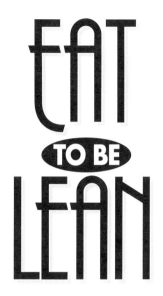

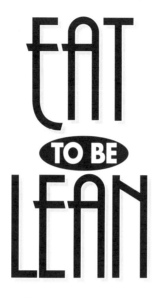

A Step-by-Step Guide to a Healthy Eating Lifestyle

Michele A. Morgan

Mainstream Publishing
P.O. Box 1252
Snohomish, WA 98291

The following trademarks appear throughout this book: Grapenuts, Shredded Wheat, Zoom, Butter Buds, Wondra, 2 - Alarm Chili Kit, Carroll Shelby Chili Mix, and Boboli.

Eat to be Lean. Copyright 1996 by Michele A. Morgan. All rights reserved. No part of this book may be reproduced in any form, or by any electronic, mechanical, or other means including information storage and retrieval systems, without permission in writing from the author, except by a reviewer, who may quote brief passages in a review. Published by Mainstream Publishing, P.O. Box 1252, Snohomish, WA 98291

Library of Congress Catalog Card number: 96-95156

ISBN: 0-9655644-0-1

Book ordering information is located at the back of the book or by contacting Mainstream Publishing, P.O. Box 1252, Snohomish, WA 98291.

Design by: Visual Graphics, Mukilteo, WA

Acknowledgments

I would like to give special thanks to Cynthia Papeman-Youll, Florence McIntyre, Tina Ruybal, Sherry Jury and Janine Houck, for their expertise, honesty, enthusiasm and dotting my "i's" and crossing my "t's".

Dedications

Dedicated to everyone who has ever asked me, "What do you eat?"
Since I could not give a short answer,
Eat to be Lean was born.

I would also like to dedicate the following pages to my best friend, lover and business partner. Thank you so much for the constant encouragement, confidence and being brave enough to taste all those experimental meals.
I love you.

TABLE OF CONTENTS

Introduction 1

I. **Simple Understandings** 5

    a) Carbohydrates 5
    b) Protein 6
    c) Fats 7
    d) How often should I eat? 8
    e) How much should I eat? 9
    f) Read Labels 9
    g) How do I make this easy on myself? 10

II. **Taking Your First Step** 11

III. **To the Market** 15

    a) Master Grocery List 17
    b) Uses and Comments 21

IV. **Never Say Never** 35

V. **Making Better Decisions** 37

    a) Food Substitutes 38
    b) Preparation Alternatives 40
    c) Baking Hints 41
    d) Restaurant Food Choices 42
    e) Taboo on the Menu 47

VI. **Lattes, Mochas, Breves and More** 51

VII. **So You Need to Gain a Few Pounds?** 55

VIII. **Exercise** 57

IX. **Menu Ideas** 59

    a) Breakfast/Brunch 60
    b) Lunch 61
    c) Dinner 62
    d) Side Dishes 63
    e) Snacks and Appetizers 64
    f) Desserts 64

X.   Recipes 65

    a) Breakfast/Brunch 68
        1) Breakfast Favorites 69
        2) Hot Cereals 71
        3) Egg Dishes 72
        4) Breakfast Potatoes 78
    b) Muffins 79
    c) Lunch 85
        1) Sandwiches 86
        2) Soups 88
    d) Dinner 90
        1) Crock Pot Dinners 92
        2) Family Favorites 94
        3) Chili 98
        4) Mexican Dishes 101
        5) Italian and Pasta Dishes 106
        6) Vegetable Dishes 110
    e) Side Dishes 112
        1) Vegetable Side Dishes 113
        2) Potato Side Dishes 115
        3) Salads 119
    f) Appetizers 121
    g) Desserts 124

Bibliography 129

Index 130

Introduction

I see it every day, the struggles of diet and exercise. People are trying desperately to take off weight and fight off signs of aging such as decreased metabolism and muscle atrophy. They are exercising regularly trying to keep their bodies fit and healthy. As co-owner of a gym and having been active in the health and fitness field for the last seventeen years, it seems the biggest hurdle to overcome is what, how and when to eat.

Finally!! A practical approach to eating that won't complicate your life or require that you be a math whiz to be successful. *Eat to be Lean* will show you how to approach eating healthy, in easy, non-scientific ways that can easily be incorporated into everyday living.

Eat to be Lean was inspired by a question that I am frequently asked, "What do you eat?" This question often comes from what people see when they look at me, a healthy, nicely musculatured, fit body. I exercise regularly and incorporate good nutrition and sensible eating into my daily life in order to maintain this level of fitness and health. The purpose of *Eat to be Lean* is to share these ideals so that you too can learn to be in control of how you eat, what you eat, and to ultimately enjoy the benefits of looking great and feeling healthy.

Like many of you, I have read all about fats, carbohydrates, proteins, sugars, calorie counting and expenditure, portion control, label reading and diets of all kinds. Many of you have probably tried a fad diet or two, maybe with success, but what happens when the diet ends? Normally, you gain back all the weight lost and more. You've studied, investigated and experimented with all of the information you've gathered and collected, but you still can't quite figure out what to do with it all. Just where and how do you start to put all this knowledge to work for you and your family? *Eat to be Lean* will show you how to create a lifestyle of eating leaner and healthier.

You'll never have to diet again. This guide will walk you through the process of preparing your food supply for cooking healthy meals and help put the knowledge you've already obtained to work for you. It will teach you how to cook lean without sacrificing flavor when preparing foods low in sugars, fats and salt.

The recipes included are not fancy or difficult to prepare. They are basic "meat and potato" meals made lean. Menus are included to save you time and take the guess work out of "What am I going to make for breakfast? Lunch? Dinner?" *Eat to be Lean* will show you that cooking is not difficult and that it is not a science which needs to be mastered by exactness in order to serve a successful meal. Cooking and baking have always been passions of mine. I have gone from a gourmet cook whose main ingredients were olive oil, real butter, garlic, cheeses and sugars, to a gourmet cook whose main ingredients are now non-stick cooking spray, onions, still lots of garlic, bell peppers, nonfat cheeses and unsweetened fruit juices. With a few simple changes and some discipline, you can prepare great tasting, healthy, well-balanced meals.

Not only will the information in *Eat to be Lean* be beneficial to people trying to lose weight, it will be just as useful to those trying to gain weight. Even though a majority of the population has little sympathy for this special group of people, gaining weight can be just as much a struggle as trying to lose weight or maintain an ideal weight ("weight" referring specifically to body fat percentage). Usually people trying to gain weight have a very low percentage of body fat and no doubt want to keep it that way as they strive to gain lean body mass. The principles described in *Eat to be Lean* may be applied to gaining weight as well. Every "body", no matter how big or small, can benefit from eating leaner and healthier.

People often believe that if they are eating foods labeled "fat free", they can consume as much of that food as they want and not gain any weight or body fat. This simply is not true, "fat free" does not mean all-you-can-eat. Eating lean consists of more than just eating foods that are low in fat. Caloric intake considerations, keeping processed sugar intake as low as possible and maintaining a good balance of protein and carbohydrates in each meal is essential. Be careful when purchasing "fat free" foods, many contain unfamiliar ingredients and high levels of sodium and sugars for added flavor.

Eat to be Lean has been divided into ten valuable chapters. Chapter I explains basic terminology and guidelines to monitor the quality of your meals to help move you closer to your nutritional goals. Chapters II and III show you how to organize and stock your kitchen pantry, taking you step-by-step toward getting your kitchen workspace in order. Chapter III shares my typical grocery list which will organize your shopping days and get you in and out of the grocery store more quickly. Chapter III also includes *Uses and Comments* in reference to the grocery store items. Here I have discussed the various ways some food items can be used. This will encourage your creativeness when it comes to customizing your own personal recipes and menu plans.

Never Say Never, Chapter IV, is a comprehensive list of foods and beverages that should not be a part of your every day meals and only allowed on occasion, quite infrequently. They are foods that are highest in fats and sugars.

In the busy lives of today, you'll find Chapter V extremely useful. *Making Better Decisions* trains you to think about eating lean whenever you prepare meals, grocery shop and dine out. It highlights the wiser alternatives you will begin making. Learn how to make any recipe leaner by studying the *Food Substitutes, Preparation Alternatives* and *Baking Hints*. Master ordering food in a restaurant by understanding different ways food can be specially prepared in *Restaurant Food Choices*. *Taboo on the Menu* describes which menu items to stay away from or have special-ordered to accommodate eating lean. A glossary of terms is provided describing the names of certain dishes and how they are prepared enabling you to make smart choices while dining out.

As the coffee craze hits the rest of America you'll need to learn how to best order that cup of Java. Chapter VI, *Lattes, Mochas, Breves and More*, familiarizes you with the most popular coffee drinks, how they are typically served and how they can be ordered to best suit your new healthy lifestyle. It also represents other popular beverages available at your favorite coffee stand or coffee cafe.

Since not everybody needs to lose a few pounds, Chapter VII sheds light on what it takes to *gain* lean body mass. Chapter VIII supports exercise, encouraging you to incorporate a complete and regular exercise program into your lifestyle.

Chapter IX contains menu ideas that will do the deciding for you when it comes to preparing your next meal. Menu selections may be chosen from six categories including *Breakfast/Brunch, Lunch, Dinner, Side Dishes, Snacks and Appetizers*, and *Desserts*. Trying to decide what to cook for the next meal, day after day, may seem quite burdensome. These menus offer good ideas enabling you to decide more quickly and will also keep you on the right track of eating lean.

Lastly, Chapter X includes a selection of my favorite recipes chosen from the menu ideas. Many of the recipes have optional ingredients and variations for preparation - in case you are short an ingredient or two, or just want a little bit different flavor than the last time. Keep in mind that you cook to please your own palate and those of your family and friends. Cooking variations are endless, which is what makes cooking and eating so pleasurable!

Learning to eat lean takes practice and discipline. You know yourself well enough to do what it takes to wean yourself away from those foods you know you shouldn't be eating, those foods too high in fat and refined sugars. Being creative with your new ingredients takes practice as well. As you become more accustomed to these new changes, eating lean will be a natural part of your everyday life, wherever you enjoy your meals. You will no longer miss the foods you are used to eating and realize that eating healthy can be very satisfying and pleasurable. I can't think of a better way to enjoy a meal than being able to eat without guilt. You won't have to worry about whether or not you are going to be able to fit into those jeans the next time you want to wear them, or panic about standing on the scale. You will be in control of the aesthetics and good health of your body.

The four meals I prepare each day are flavorful and always have a good balance of protein and carbohydrates. Each meal is extremely low in fat and sugar and the portions are kept in proportion to my physical size and needs. Exercising regularly, eating four to five small meals daily and eating lean, well-balanced meals can keep you healthy, trim and confident too.

I hope you find *Eat to be Lean* a very valuable tool in making positive changes toward a new lifestyle of living and eating healthy.

BON APPETITE'

Simple Understandings

Let us begin by discussing some very basic information about food and answering commonly asked questions.

Many people do not eat well-balanced meals because they are unaware of which foods supply carbohydrates, proteins and fats, or any combination thereof. For example, women tend to lack protein in their diet, going meal after meal with out a single gram. Men, on the other hand, tend to eat too much protein and lack important carbohydrates such as grains, fruits and vegetables. Both extremes can lead to weight gain, just the thing most of us are trying to avoid. Explained below are ideal sources of carbohydrates, proteins and fats and the purposes they serve.

Carbohydrates

The body's main source of energy comes from carbohydrates. The carbohydrates listed below should constitute 55-60% of your daily caloric intake, and in the same proportions in each meal. Healthy choice foods high in carbohydrates include:

Fruits
Vegetables
Grains: Barley, corn, oats, rice, rye and wheat.
    Foods made from grains: Breads, pasta, cereals, tortillas, popcorn, bulgur.
Potatoes

Carbohydrates are also supplied through sugars that come from fruits. Fruit offers a great source of vitamins, minerals, fiber, and the healthiest form of sugar. Refined sugars include white table sugar, brown sugar, and corn syrup.

These sugars contribute to obesity, tooth decay, mineral depletion, diabetes, arthritis and other health risks. Honey and molasses contain a few more nutrients than refined sugars but should still be consumed in moderation.

Refined carbohydrates such as white flour, white rice and refined sugars are processed so greatly that they have lost virtually all nutritional value. The manufacturer attempts to put back (enrich) the nutrients lost in processing, however, leaving the finished product lacking in nutritional quality. That is one of the reasons it is best not to consume foods made with "enriched" white or whole wheat flour. It is difficult to find certain bread items made with 100% whole grain flours. Bagels, flour tortillas, crackers, burger buns, pizza dough, biscuit and pancake mix all contain varying amounts of enriched flours. In these cases, purchase brands that use whole wheat flour, whether it is enriched or not. Some bread items include whole wheat and white flours. You will benefit from the higher fiber content provided by wheat and other whole grain flours. Loaves of bread can easily be found made with 100% whole wheat, or stone ground whole wheat flours. If you make bread at home use 100% whole wheat or other whole grain flours. Multi-grain breads are good but may contain too much fat, read the labels.

Proteins

Proteins provide the building blocks for all tissues of the human body. All bodily functions, including rate of metabolism, muscle growth, water balance, production of hair, nails, skin and blood, and proper functioning of the heart, brain and internal organs are all dependent on sufficient amounts and proper sources of protein. Proteins should constitute 30-35% of your daily caloric intake, and in the same proportions in each meal. Choose proteins from the following food groups:

Eggs (whites only) or egg substitutes made from eggs.
Dairy Products: Nonfat - cheeses (hard, cottage, cream), milk, yogurt, sour cream.
Seafood.
Poultry: Turkey and chicken (skinless).
Meats: Beef, pork, lamb, veal.
Legumes: Peas, lentils, beans.
　Types of beans: Kidney, pinto, white, navy, black.
Soybean products.

Nuts and seeds are also sources of protein, but due to their high fat content, should be eaten infrequently and in small quantities. Some soybean products may be high in fat, read labels carefully.

Common fish that contain more than 3 grams of fat per three ounce serving include carp, catfish, eel, herring, mackerel, salmon, shark, swordfish and trout. Choose to eat these fish only occasionally. Shellfish are low in fat but contain high amounts of cholesterol, these too should be eaten in moderation and only occasionally.

Meats fall into two categories, muscle meats and organ meats (liver, kidneys, hearts, brains, glands/sweetbreads and tongue). Meats (including poultry) and dairy products are the most complete forms of protein. The leanest cuts of beef are rounds and loins; eye of round, round tip, top round, top loin, sirloin and tenderloin. The light meat of poultry is leaner than the dark portions.

Fats

Fat contains the greatest amount of energy per gram. That is why the body stores anything you eat in excess as fat. If you ingest more food (energy) than the body needs to function, the excess, whether it is proteins, carbohydrates or fats, is stored as fat waiting to be used at another time. Fat serves many useful purposes and includes essential fatty acids enabling the body to function correctly and efficiently. That is why it is unsafe to be on a completely no-fat diet. Our bodies do need certain fats, but only in small quantities.

The two different types of fat making the headlines today are saturated and unsaturated. Unsaturated fats are found in liquid form and are derived from vegetables. Saturated fats are usually found in a solid state and come mostly from animals. Unsaturated fats are preferable. There are enough fats found naturally in foods that adding extra fats to foods is unnecessary and should be avoided whenever possible. Fats should constitute no more than 10-15% of your daily caloric intake, and in the same proportions in each meal. More often than not, avoid eating foods with three or more grams of fat per serving. Often serving sizes are very small and people tend to eat more that one serving at a time. This can cause the total fat intake to be quite high.

Read the nutrition labels! Do your best to eat foods where no more than 20% of the total calories, per serving come from fat. Reading labels can be tricky. In fact, most food manufacturers round-down the total number of calories and fat grams per serving. One gram of carbohydrates equals four calories. One gram of protein also equals four calories, and one gram of fat lends nine calories. If a serving size contains a total of 100 calories, and the total fat grams per serving is three, that equates to 27 fat calories, meaning one serving contains 27% fat (three grams of fat multiplied by nine calories per gram, divided by the totals number of calories, 100, times 100 equals 27%). See the example in Chapter II, *Taking Your First Step*, for further clarification. The other sixty-three calories are divided between carbohydrates and proteins. Following is a list of some common high fat food items, choose to eat these foods only in moderation and with very little frequency:

Avocado
Beef
Butter/margarine
Cheeses *
Chocolate
Dairy products *
Egg yolks
Mayonnaise

Nuts/nut butters
Oils
Olives
Salad dressings: oil/mayonnaise based
Salami
Sausages/bacon
Shortening

* Products made with whole milk.

For a more complete listing of high-fat foods refer to Chapter IV, *Never Say Never*.

How often should I eat?

It is better to eat 4-5 smaller, well-balanced meals throughout the day rather than 1-2 larger meals. Most people should go no longer than 4-5 hours without food. If eating this frequently is too difficult to fit into your schedule, eat no less than three average-sized meals and a snack in-between meals. A snack is something small in quantity and should be low in fats, sugars and calories; unbuttered popcorn, 6-8 ounces of yogurt, a piece of fruit, vegetables, hard-boiled egg whites, cottage cheese. One of the keys to weight loss and staying lean is to have a high metabolism. Your metabolism is something you can control, to a large degree, from eating and exercising. Each time you consume a meal your metabolism increases during digestion. When your body gets used to eating every 4-5 hours your metabolism automatically increases during these times, overall remaining higher throughout the day. Exercise also increases metabolism, not only during active exercise but for a couple of hours afterwards.

One of the best ways to gain weight (body fat) is to skip meals. If you deprive your body of fuel (food) your metabolism drops to conserve energy. Your body will store much of what you do decide to eat as fat thinking that it isn't going to be fueled again for quite sometime. This is why you will often hear overweight people confess that they don't eat much at all. They are right, most of them don't. This is one of their biggest problems. You must get your body on a consistent eating routine to increase metabolism and decrease body fat storage.

How much should I eat?

How much you can eat depends largely on whether or not you are trying to gain or lose weight. It also depends on your metabolic rate, lean muscle mass and activity level. It can be very scientific, but let's keep is simple.

Most people who are trying to lose weight know how much is too much. No second helpings, smaller portions, no skipping of meals and a good balance of proteins and carbohydrates is a great place to start (55-60% carbohydrates, 30-35% proteins and 10-15% fats). You cannot eat an endless amount of "fat free" food just because it is fat free. The same applies to sugar free foods. Calories are still the most crucial element in losing weight. The amount of calories eaten must be less than the amount of calories expended. Become more active, exercise regularly to expend more calories.

For gaining weight you must eat, eat and eat some more. Even if you think you already eat like a horse, start eating like an army. If you have to, set your alarm for sometime in the middle of the night and eat again. Be sure what you eat is mostly lean so the weight you do put on won't just be fat. Eat high calorie foods, a lot of snacks and don't skip meals. If you are already extremely lean and don't have a tendency to store body fat, you may indulge more often in higher fat foods. Try a weight gain drink as a snack (see recipe in Chapter VII). You may get very tired of eating all the time, but you *must* in order to obtain your goals. Balanced meals are just as important when trying to gain weight. You need a lot of carbohydrates for energy and sufficient amounts of protein for growth. Read Chapter VII for more detailed information about gaining weight.

Read Labels:

In order to understand how much to eat and what to eat, you must learn to read labels and get to know the contents of the foods you are eating. It is the only way to fully understand how many calories you are consuming and the ratios of carbohydrates, proteins and fats provided for each serving. If you are not already familiar with the calorie content of foods, you may have to start tallying the total number of calories you are consuming each day to get the true picture. This will no doubt give you a direction as far as knowing whether you are eating too much or too little. To prevent weight gain due to under eating, the average woman should not eat less than

1,200 - 1,400 calories per day, and the average man should consume no less than 1,400-1,800 calories per day. There are many factors that figure into these amounts, but these are the basic guidelines. The more physically active you are and the more lean body mass you have, the more food you can eat on a daily basis without experiencing weight gain. Eating less than the stated amounts for men and women can lead to weight gain very easily for most people. On the other hand, people who have a difficult time gaining weight, will only continue to lose weight if they do not fuel their bodies sufficiently.

Sodium is also an important bit of information found on nutrition labels. With so many foods being made "fat free" these days, unfortunately, the sodium content has been increased to help flavor these foods. Avoid foods with more that 500mg of sodium per serving, of course, the lower the sodium content the better. Processed sugars have been added for the same flavoring purposes. Read the list of ingredients to find added sugars. If sugar, corn syrup or high fructose corn syrup is listed first, second or third the sugars are too high. Exceptions may be barbecue sauce and salad dressings which are used in very small amounts.

Start to educate yourself about the foods and beverages you are consuming so you can begin to make smart and healthy decisions for your body.

How do I make this easy on myself?

So you don't want to count calories, measure food portions or calculate protein, carbohydrate and fat grams. I can't blame you, and that is why I don't.

Choose foods listed earlier in this chapter under "Carbohydrates" and "Proteins", in low fat or nonfat form if available. Avoid those foods listed under "Fats" and in the list provided in Chapter IV, *Never Say Never*. When you serve yourself a meal, make sure the food fits on the plate without spilling over or mounding into sky-scraper formations. Make sure you have a serving of protein and one or two servings of carbohydrates, preferably from the fruits, vegetables, and grain categories. Take it easy on the added fats, many foods, especially proteins, contain low levels of natural fats. Discipline will be your biggest challenge. Remember your goals and make good health a priority.

Taking Your First Step

Before taking the first step it is advantageous to get yourself into a positive frame of mind. Following are a few things to think about to get you moving toward a productive mode of change.

Many aspects of our lives are governed by outside sources. Work, family, time restraints, deadlines, rules, regulations, weather and other obligations seem to dictate a great deal of our day-to-day lives. Deciding what you eat may be one of the only things in your life you have full reign over. Take advantage of this and use it to be in control of how you look and feel. People are most productive and happy when they are confident about their appearance and feel strong and healthy. When you look good, you feel invincible.

There are several ways to begin taking charge of what you eat. You can start by controlling the type of food you eat by choosing foods and beverages low in fats and sugars. The amount of food you eat can be controlled by serving yourself smaller portions and to stop eating when you feel the first signs of fullness. Stop eating whether or not there is food left on your plate. The quality of your meals can be maintained by making sure you have adequate portions of carbohydrates and proteins (refer to Chapter I). Drink water with a majority of your meals instead of milk, juice, soda, tea, coffee or alcoholic beverages.

If you find that you are often discouraged and depressed about how you look and feel, keep this in mind: *If you begin today to make positive changes towards a healthy lifestyle, you won't get any worse than you are right now. This is as bad as it gets, you will only improve from this point forward. Results and improvement begin when you do.* Let this encourage you to take the first step towards a beautiful and healthy body. Ask yourself these questions, "How seriously do I want to look good, feel great and feel confident? Do I want to live a healthy lifestyle? Do I want to have a higher quality of life?" If you want it, you can have it. If you want it bad enough, you will succeed. You are in complete control of this aspect of your life. With your positive frame of mind, and strong will, you are ready to take the first step.

Before rushing to the grocery store to stock up on all the healthy food you can find, there is one thing that you *must* do first. This is where you begin to transform your food inventory by getting rid of those food items and ingredients that don't belong in your new lifestyle. If you do not take this first step, it may be too easy to falter back to the old ways of eating. First begin by taking the time and energy to revamp your kitchen cupboards, refrigerator, pantry, laundry room, garage, storage shed, under your bed or any other place you might store food. Now depending on whether or not your home is prepared for a natural disaster, this task could take anywhere from thirty minutes to two days. My own cupboards are usually more like Old Mother Hubbard's cupboards so this didn't take me quite as long.

Before beginning this task supply yourself with some empty boxes or bags. You will also need to decide where the food you are getting rid of will be disbursed. Food banks, homeless shelters, food drives, women's shelters or other family members and friends would be great places to donate this food.

What you need to do is go through every single food item in your home and remove those items that are too high in fats and sugars. Some basic guidelines to begin with would be to eliminate anything containing more than 3.0 grams of fat per serving. A stricter guideline would be to eliminate those foods whose fat percent per serving is more than 20%. If the fat percent per serving is not listed on the label, you will need to calculate it yourself. Don't confuse the percent of fat per serving with the "% Daily Value", which is commonly found on labels. Multiply the number of fat grams per serving by nine. Take that total and divide it by the number of calories per serving, then multiply that number by 100. This will give you the percent of fat per serving. See the following example:

Amount per serving
Calories 163
Calories from fat 27

Total Fat   3 g. x 9 calories/gram = 27 total fat calories
Total Carbohydrates 25 g. x 4 calories/gram = 100 total carbohydrate calories
Total Proteins   9 g. x 4 calories/gram = <u>36</u> total protein calories
                                   163 total calories

3 g. fat x 9 calories/gram = 27 fat calories, divided by 163 calories per serving x 100 = **16.5 %** fat per serving.

Anything that has sugar, corn syrup, high fructose corn syrup or molasses listed first, second or third on the list of ingredients, must also be eliminated, as well as, anything containing more than 500 mg. of sodium per serving. Exceptions to this rule are condiments such as catsup, pickles, mayonnaise, barbecue sauce, low fat and nonfat salad dressings, as well as some seasoning packets. These items should always be used in small quantities, leaving the amount of sugars and sodium insignificant to your daily food intake.

The following phrase is extremely important to remember, *if it's not there, you can't eat it.* If the cookies aren't in the cupboard, you can't eat them. If there is no candy in the candy dish, you can't eat it. If there is no butter in the refrigerator, you can't smother your baked potato in it or spread it on toast. If the ice cream isn't in the freezer, you'll have to go without. Of course you can always hop in your car and go down to the store if you absolutely can't be without, but more than likely you won't make the effort.

At this point you might be thinking, "Yeah, right!" You may have kids of varying ages and a spouse not interested at all in eating healthier. They are quite happy with how they look, how they feel and what they eat. If this is the case you have alternatives.

If you are in control of most of the cooking and grocery shopping, the changes you make will benefit all family members. You may have to set up one section in the kitchen cupboards, pantry and refrigerator/freezer that is designated for those snacks or food items that you will no longer be eating, but others in the family will still want to indulge in. Help your family to make the transition by keeping minimal amounts of sweets, snacks and high fat foods on hand. The same logic works for them, *if it's not there, they won't eat it.* Learn to replace those high fat, high sugar foods with such substitutes as fruit juice popsicles, fruit sorbets, fat free pretzels, popcorn that can be air-popped and keep more fruit available to help satisfy the sweet cravings.

Depending on when your next shopping day is, it might be best to begin by replacing food items that are consumed more frequently. For instance, milk, bread, cereal and condiments are used quite often and should be replaced right away. If you won't be shopping for a couple of days or so, start by eliminating all of the dessert goodies and snacks such as cookies, candy, ice cream and chips. If you simply cannot go cold turkey, without sweets or snacks, substitute these items with something more healthy before you discard them (and think again about what your goals are.) Continue this process until your whole kitchen and all food storage spaces are free from foods that should no longer be there.

I can just picture you standing there in the middle of this newly revamped kitchen. The cupboards are open exposing their bareness and you are standing there looking in the refrigerator trying to figure out what to eat. It all seems so foreign, now what do you do? It becomes overwhelming and you start to panic. You begin to hunt for your car keys, grab your wallet and head for the nearest fast food restaurant. **STOP!** Don't panic! Change is difficult but you *can* do this.

Now that your cupboards are bare and you have a fresh start, continue on to Chapter III, *To the Market* for guidance in grocery shopping.

To the Market

The following grocery list was designed to make your shopping easier and quicker. The items listed are the main ingredients you will now be using in everyday cooking. The *Master Grocery List* includes everything for a fully stocked kitchen. In bold print, are food items I use most often. They are the staple ingredients you need to begin cooking and eating lean. Something can always be made with these few items on hand. You will find that many of these ingredients need to be replenished on your next trip to the grocery store. The asterisked items are ingredients I keep stocked at all times. They are mostly condiments, herbs and spices, baking ingredients and other common staple foods. You may already have many of these items on hand. They are the necessary tools to flavoring, thickening, particular cooking methods, and are the basic ingredients to many recipes.

If you have already taken a peak ahead, don't be alarmed by the extent of the *Master Grocery List*! Not everything on this list needs to be purchased at once depending on your tastes and needs. It goes beyond the basics to make meal planning simple. After completing *The First Step*, and before going to the grocery store, use the *Master Grocery List* as a checklist for food items you already have in stock and to get a better idea of what you will be shopping for. Several copies of this list can be made for your personal use by circling items you will be picking up on your next visit to the grocery store. I post one on my refrigerator door and circle the items I get low on, run out of, or will be needing in a particular recipe being prepared in the near future.

Not all the foods listed will appeal to your taste and there may be certain herbs, spices, vegetables, or fruits you like that are not mentioned. Feel free to venture outside of this list and please your own palate, making sure to stay within the guidelines of low-to-no fats, refined sugars and sodium. Some items may be ignored altogether, for instance, if you know you won't be doing any baking, many of those items listed under Baking Spices/Ingredients need not be considered.

This list serves as a guideline for ideas and begins to make you think about foods you don't normally purchase. Studying this list and purchasing these items will make the question "What should I have to eat?" much easier to answer.

Before becoming too overwhelmed with the grocery list, and before omitting any items, be sure to review *Uses and Comments*. This section contains various uses for most of the food items listed, along with very helpful hints to assist you in making better product choices, and enable you to narrow down your shopping list. Reviewing the *Menu Ideas* and *Recipes* in Chapters IX and X, respectively, may also furnish you with ideas about what foods you will want to start with. As stated in *The First Step*, restocking your kitchen can be done in small steps by replacing a little bit at a time, meal-by-meal if necessary.

I grocery shop about once every 5-8 days, with an occasional "run in" for unfreckled bananas, eggs or milk. My shopping routine follows the same pattern of isle browsing each time. Since I purchase the same items week after week, shopping has become very predictable and takes very little time. With some getting used to and breaking away from old shopping habits, you too will become more familiar with the set-up and food selection of your local grocery store. You will be going to the store knowing what you need, where to find it and be in and out of there very quickly.

MASTER GROCERY LIST

BREAD - BAKERY

100% Whole wheat, sliced
Burger Buns, whole grain

Bagels - water made
Pizza shell

DAIRY

Nonfat milk - Carton and dry
Evaporated skim milk
Nonfat sour cream
Eggs or egg substitutes

Nonfat cottage cheese
Nonfat yogurt
Nonfat, grated cheeses

MEAT (BEEF, PORK)

Eye of round roast
Boneless beef ribs
London broil
Beef stew meat, extra lean

Pork loin roast
Boneless pork chops
Boneless pork ribs
Ham, extra lean, whole or sliced

POULTRY

Ground turkey breast
Whole turkey breast
Smoked turkey breast

Turkey breast tenderloins
Chicken breast, boneless, skinless

FISH

Tuna
Snapper
Flounder and soles
Ling cod

Orange Roughy
Halibut
Swordfish ♦
Shark ♦

♦ Fat content is slightly higher than 3 grams per serving, eat only in moderation.

MISCELLANEOUS MEATS

Chunk light chicken (water packed)
Chunk light tuna (water packed)
Lunch meats - roast beef, ham, turkey

Canadian bacon
Turkey bacon ■

■ Use only as a topping, fat percentage is too high to eat as a side dish.

PRODUCE - FRUIT

Fresh or frozen
Seasonal fruit (except avocados)
Bananas
Berries
Peaches
Grapes
Apples

Packaged
Raisins
Applesauce, unsweetened
Pineapple, in its own juice
Sliced pears or peaches, it their own juice

PRODUCE - VEGETABLES

Fresh
Onions - White, green, yellow
Bell peppers - Green, red, yellow or orange
Potatoes - Russet, red, white
Tomatoes
Mushrooms
Green leaf lettuce
Cabbage
Squashes
Garlic *
Celery

Fresh or frozen
Carrots
String beans
Corn
Broccoli
Spinach
Vegetable mixes

CEREALS

Cold
Whole grain - wheat, corn, oat, rice
Shredded Wheat
Grapenuts

Hot
Oats
Whole wheat - *Zoom*
Mixed grains

CANNED FOODS

Beans
Refried - fat free
Pinto, seasoned
Black /Negro
Pork and Beans
Kidney

Broths
Chicken (low sodium)
Beef
Vegetable

Tomato
Stewed -variously seasoned
Paste
Sauce

Chunky sauces - variously seasoned
Spaghetti sauce
Marinara

Miscellaneous
Pumpkin
Water chestnuts, sliced

Green chilies, diced

OTHER HIGH ENERGY CARBOHYDRATES
Pasta
Corn or flour tortillas
  (made with no fats)

Brown or wild **rice**
Stuffing mix

CONDIMENTS
Fat free mayonnaise *
Fresh salsa *
Barbecue sauce *
Mustard *

Catsup
Nonfat salad dressing
Pickles and relish, sweet or dill

BEVERAGES
Unsweetened fruit juices
Tomato/vegetable juice

Apple juice concentrate

SPICE CABINET

Baking Spices
Cinnamon *
Vanilla/Maple **extracts** *

Nutmeg
Allspice

Herbs and Spices
Garlic powder *
Italian herb blends *
Poultry seasoning *
Chili powder *
No-salt blends *
Cumin

Onion powder
Paprika
Pepper
Dill
Cajun blend

Seasoning Packets
Taco/chicken taco
Spaghetti
Burrito

Beef marinade
Stew
Chili - *2-Alarm Chili Kit* or
  Carroll Shelbys Chili Mix

SNACKS
Popcorn - air popped
No-oil baked chips

Fruit popsicles
Pretzels

MISCELLANEOUS STAPLE ITEMS AND BAKING INGREDIENTS

Non-stick vegetable cooking spray *
Wondra **- gravy thickener ***
Bread crumbs - plain or seasoned
Fruit spreads *
Whole wheat flour *
Cornstarch
Baking powder *
Reduced fat biscuit mix *

Butter Buds
Whole wheat pancake
  mix
Cornmeal *
Artificial sweetener
Wine vinegar
Syrup, sugar free
Tapioca

* Items I keep stocked at all times.

Comments and Uses

Food Item	Uses	Comments
Breads		
100% Whole wheat bread	French toast, toast, burger buns, sandwiches, homemade croutons, as a side dish with meals.	Choose bread products made with 100% whole wheat or stone ground whole wheat flour. Burger buns are hard to find made with 100% whole wheat flour. Buy buns made with whole wheat or oat grain flour to ensure more fiber and vitamin content, even if the flour is enriched.
Bagels	Breakfast toast, sandwich bread, snack.	There are water-made bagels and egg-made bagels. Water-made bagels usually contain little or no fat, they would be your best choice.
Dairy		
Nonfat milk	In cereals, mashed potatoes, muffins, biscuits, or to drink with meals.	If you don't think you can handle going straight to nonfat milk in the carton, try preparing milk from instant nonfat dry milk mix. Milk made in this manner tends to have a richer flavor, making it easier to wean yourself away from milks higher in fat. Soon you will be able to enjoy regularly processed nonfat milk in cartons.
Evaporated skim milk	Gravies, cream soups, mashed potatoes, baking recipes, weight-gain drink and pumpkin porridge.	In recipes, use evaporated skim milk undiluted. Mixed with equal parts water makes regular strength milk.

Food Item	Uses	Comments
Eggs	In breakfast recipes, baking recipes, meatloaf/meatballs, egg salad sandwiches. Also used as an ingredient in coating fish, pork and chicken dishes for main course meals.	Use the egg whites only. If this is too drastic of a change, start with cutting down on the number of yolks you use, for example, in a three-egg omelette, or scrambled eggs, include only one yolk. In recipes calling for eggs, substitute one whole egg with two egg whites.
Yogurt, nonfat	Dressings, dips, fruit topping, snack, side dish and in weight-gain drink.	Try different brands until you find one you like. They differ in taste, texture and quantity.
Cottage cheese, nonfat	Baked potato topping, layered in lasanga, snack, side dish.	Read label for sodium content, stay under 500 mg per serving. The flavor of nonfat cottage cheese has improved tremendously over the years.
Sour cream, nonfat	Baked potato topping, in quiche, potato salad, Mexican food dishes.	Blend with small amounts of milk for a creamier texture.
Hard cheeses, nonfat	Mexican food dishes, quiche, omelettes, lasanga, pizza, Philly-style steak sandwich, salad and baked potato topping, in twice-baked potatoes and potato skin appetizers.	There are a variety of nonfat grated cheeses available. Some have combined flavors such as jack and cheddar.

Meat (Beef and Pork)

Purchase the leanest cuts of meats available; round and loins. Purchase the leanest of the rounds and loins by selecting the least marbled cuts available at the meat counter.

Food Item	Uses	Comments
London Broil	As a main course. Leftovers as steak sandwiches, beef stroganoff, burritos, minced in soups, sliced for breakfast and added to omelettes.	
Eye of round beef roast	As a main course. Leftovers as barbecue beef sandwiches, beef burritos, beef tacos, tostadas, nachos or added to soup.	
Pork loin roast	As a main course. Leftovers as barbecue pork sandwiches, pork burritos, pork tacos or tostadas.	
Ham	As a main course, sliced in sandwiches, breakfast meat, omelettes, quiche filling, pizza topping, minced in soups or on salads, baked potato topping.	Purchase lean ham, 97% - 99% fat free. To be consumed in moderation due to high sodium content. Do not buy canned hams.

Poultry

Food Item	Uses	Comments
Ground turkey breast	In any recipe calling for ground beef, substitute with lean ground turkey breast. Spaghetti meat sauce, meatloaf/meatballs, chili, chili casserole, lasagna, burgers, manicotti, stuffed bell peppers, egg hash and Mexican food dishes.	Look for ground turkey breast without the skin, 99% fat free. Some ground turkey includes the skin making it approximately 93% fat free. Sometimes I mix the two for a moister texture.

Food Item	Uses	Comments
Whole turkey breast or breast tenderloins	As a main course. Leftovers as sliced turkey or turkey salad sandwiches, add to soups, stroganoff, in Mexican food dishes.	I have often found the whole turkey breast packaged for sale. Ask your butcher for availability. Remove skin from whole turkey breast before cooking.
Smoked turkey breast	Diced in omelettes or sliced as breakfast meat, sandwiches, on salads.	Look for 97% - 99% fat free smoked turkey breasts. Consume in moderation due to high sodium content.
Chicken breast	As a main course. Tacos, burritos, nachos, tostadas, chicken salad sandwiches, stroganoff, add to soup.	Remove skin before cooking.
Fish		**Purchase fresh fish when available; fresh/frozen or previously frozen is the next best choice.**
Orange Roughy Ling Cod Flounder/Soles Snapper	These fish are great for broiling, steaming, pan frying or baking. They can be lightly breaded or seasoned.	
Halibut Swordfish Shark Tuna	These fish are great for barbecuing, kebabs, broiling or baking.	Since these fish are a little high in fat, eat only in moderation.

Food Item	Uses	Comments
Miscellaneous Meats, Poultry and Fish		
Lunch meats		Purchase meats 98% - 99% fat free. Consume in moderation due to high sodium content. Roast beef, ham, turkey breast and chicken breast are the leanest of the lunch meats. Purchase meats you can see, like from a deli counter so that you can visually inspect the leanness and authenticity. Look for slices of real meat, not pressed or processed.
Chicken, canned	Chicken salad sandwiches, in soups, on salads.	Purchase chicken that is packed in water; white meat only.
Ham slices Canadian bacon Turkey bacon	Sandwiches, in salads, pizza topping, breakfast meat, in omelettes, add to soups and beans, on burgers, baked potato topping.	Sodium is sometimes high. Consume in moderation. Use turkey bacon in small amounts, as in a topping.
Canned tuna	Sandwiches, salads.	Purchased tuna packed in water. Chunk light tuna is lower in fat than canned albacore tuna.
Produce - Fruits (Fresh or Frozen)		
Bananas Berries, Peaches Apples, Raisins	In muffins, snacks, desserts, toppings for cereal, pancakes, French toast and waffles, in weight-gain drink.	**Purchase fresh fruits when available. When buying frozen or canned fruits, make sure there is no added sugar.**

Miscellaneous Fruits

	Uses	Comments
Pineapple	Pizza topping, in kebabs, fruit salads, snack, top cottage cheese, in omelettes.	Purchase pineapple, and other canned fruits, sweetened in its own juice; no added sugar or corn syrups.
Applesauce	In muffins, on pancakes, waffles or French toast, as a side dish, on hot cereal, in baking recipes as a substitute for oils and shortenings.	Purchase unsweetened applesauce.
Fruit spreads	On toast, pancakes, waffles or French toast, add to hot cereals to flavor and sweeten.	Fruit spreads are jams and jellies sweetened with fruit juices instead of sugar.

Produce - Vegetables

When purchasing frozen and canned vegetables, read labels carefully. Many brands are high in sodium and have added sugars and fats.

Fresh Vegetables

	Uses	Comments
Onions - White, yellow, green Bell peppers - Green, yellow, red Garlic	Chili, spaghetti, manicotti, burgers, meatloaf/meatballs, salads, pizza topping, roasting, crock pot cooking, Mexican and Italian recipes, rice dishes, sautéed, pasta primavera.	Use these ingredients in most of your cooking to enhance flavor. You will want to always have these on hand.
Carrots	In stews, soups, salads, snack, side dish.	Thin carrots and baby carrots are usually sweeter and less bitter.

Food Item	Uses	Comments
Mushrooms	On burgers, in spaghetti, omelettes, sandwiches, pizza topping, in salads, sautéed, pasta primavera, stroganoff and quiche filling.	To make slicing mushrooms a breeze, use an egg slicer. Mushrooms can be bought pre-sliced, which is very handy and saves time.
Potatoes - Russet, red, white	Mashed, baked, twice-baked, French fried, hash browns, breakfast side dish, added to stew and soups, potato salad, egg hash.	Purchase potatoes that are firm and don't have any eyes (roots) growing from them.
Cabbage	In Mexican food recipes instead of lettuce, coleslaw, stuffed cabbage rolls, in salads, on sandwiches.	
Celery	Crock pot cooking, stuffing/dressing, in omelettes, snack, salads and in tuna, egg, chicken or turkey salad sandwiches.	
Frozen Vegetables		**Frozen vegetables are great time-savers, pick what you like. Make sure there are no added fats or sugars.**
Corn	Chili casserole, manicotti filling, stuffed bell peppers, side dish, add to cornbread.	Frozen corn is the most convenient to use in most recipes.
Spinach	Manicotti filling, omelettes, dinner	Chopped spinach is easier to work with than whole-

Food Item	Uses	Comments
	side dish, quiche filling, layered in lasagna.	leaf spinach.
Potatoes	French fries, hash browns.	Purchase fat free frozen potato products. Read the labels, there are some brands that contain zero grams of fat or less than one gram of fat per serving.

Cereals

Cold

Bran cereals	Muffin ingredient, breakfast meal, sprinkled on salads, in weight-gain drink. Bran flaked cereals can be crushed, seasoned and used for fish and poultry coatings.	Eat cereals made from whole grains; oats, barley wheat, rice, rye and corn. Choose cereals with no added fat or sugar and low in sodium. Topping cereal with fruit tastes great and adds sweetness. My personal favorites are *Shredded Wheat* and *Grapenuts*.

Hot

Oats	Use oats in meatloaf/meatballs instead of bread. Add to pancake, waffle and muffin batters and pumpkin cookie dough.	Rolled oats have a chewier texture than quick oats. Buying your oats from the bulk food section of the grocery store (if available) can save money.

Common Canned Foods

Beans

Kidney	Chili, chili casserole, salads, Mexican	These are available fat free and some can be found

Food Item	Uses	Comments
Black/Negro Pinto Chili beans, seasoned	food dishes, lunch side dish, soups.	with low sodium, compare labels.
Refried	Mexican food dishes; burritos, quesadillas, tacos, tostadas, bean dip and as a side dish.	Now available fat free and in an array of flavors. Compare brands, sodium content differs greatly.
Broths		
Chicken Beef Vegetable	Rice, gravies, crock pot cooking, roasting, basting, sautéeing, and soups.	Buy low sodium broths if available. Most are fat free or very low in fat.
Tomato		
Stewed	Chili, chili casserole, spaghetti meat sauce, chicken recipes, soups, meatloaf/meatballs, stuffed manicotti, chicken or turkey stroganoff, Mexican and Italian food dishes.	These products are available in a variety of seasonings; Italian, Mexican, chili and garden. Keep various flavors on hand to enhance different dishes. Make sure there are no added fats and sugars. Choose low sodium whenever possible.
Paste and sauces	Spaghetti sauce, chili casserole, turkey chili, manicotti, soup, stuffed cabbage rolls, stuffed bell peppers.	Purchase low sodium when available. Make sure there are no added sugars.
Miscellaneous Canned Foods		
Pumpkin	Pancakes, waffles, muffins, hot	The pumpkin porridge is a real favorite with kids.

Food item	Uses	Comments
	breakfast porridge, cookies, weight-gain drink.	See recipe.
Water chestnuts	Chinese food recipes, sauté, salads, add to rice dishes, meatloaf/meatballs, sandwiches.	Buy them already sliced to save time.
Green chilies	Chili casserole, omelette topping, nachos, tostadas, burritos, bean dip.	Make it easy on yourself, buy diced chilies.

Other High-Carbohydrate Foods

Food item	Uses	Comments
Pasta	Spaghetti, manicotti, pasta primavera, pasta salad and lasagna.	Pasta comes in many shapes and flavors. The gourmet pastas are sometimes high in fat. Some pastas are made with no egg yolks, which are a good choice. Personal preference will help you to choose a pasta; angel hair, linguini, rotini, fettuccine, spaghetti. The flavors among the different shapes are similar unless they are made with such ingredients as spinach, red pepper, dill, basil, garlic or sun-dried tomatoes. You may have to experiment with the different flavors. Just be aware of the fat content, an ounce of pasta isn't that much. Whenever possible, purchase pasta made from whole grains.

Food Item	Uses	Comments
Rice	Rice pancakes, side dish, Mexican or Spanish rice, burritos, veggie rice cakes, stuffed bell peppers.	There is a wide variety of packaged, seasoned rices available, many with no added fat. Omit the butter or margarine when preparing to keep fat grams low. Unseasoned brown rice or brown/wild rice mixtures, can be enhanced by substituting the water with broth. If making rice for breakfast rice cakes, use brown rice made with water. Wild rice, which is really a grass seed, is the most nutritious of all "rices", brown rice is a close second. Wild rice should be mixed with brown rice to make digestion easier.
Tortillas - corn or flour	Tacos, tostadas, burritos, quesadillas or make into chips.	Choose corn and flour tortillas made without lard, vegetable shortening or other fats. There are whole wheat flour tortillas available.
Stuffing/dressing mix	As a side dish, in meatloaf/meatballs, in turkey burger patties, as croutons for salad.	Look for dressing mixes with no added fat and low in sodium.

Condiments

Food Item	Uses	Comments
Fat free mayonnaise	On sandwiches and burgers, dips and salad dressings, for making tartar sauce, and in tuna, egg, chicken and turkey salad sandwiches.	

Food Item	Uses	Comments
Relishes	On burgers, in tartar sauce and in tuna, egg, chicken and turkey salad sandwiches.	
Barbecue sauce	Meatloaf/meatballs, barbecued meats and poultry, barbecue beef and pork sandwiches, add to canned beans, flavor egg hash.	When possible, purchase sauce low in sugar. Read labels and look for sugar, corn syrup or high fructose corn syrup to be listed at least third on the list of ingredients. There are many different flavors available. You may want to look in the health food section for low sugar, low sodium barbecue sauces.
Fresh salsa	Mexican food dishes, top potatoes, omelettes and fish, baked-chip dip.	There are many different salsas available made from fresh ingredients, with no added fats and very low in sodium. Look in the deli section for the freshest made salsas. They are all seasoned differently, try various brands until you find one you like.

Beverages

Food Item	Uses	Comments
Fruit juices	Flavor fruit salads, make fruit glaze, use in dessert recipes.	Purchase ready-made and juice concentrates that have no added sugar.

Miscellaneous Staple Items and Baking Ingredients

Food Item	Uses	Comments
Artificial sweetener	Muffin recipes, on cereal.	It is wise not to choose artificial sweeteners that contain saccharine. Using artificial sweeteners is

Food Item	Uses	Comments
Biscuit mix	Biscuits, dumplings, shortcake.	a personal choice to make. Use in moderation. Purchase a reduced fat biscuit mix.
Bread crumbs	Meatloaf/meatballs, coating for fish, pork and poultry, sprinkle on salads.	You can purchase plain or seasoned breadcrumbs. Compare brands for lowest fat content.
Butter Buds	Season potatoes, vegetables, popcorn.	May be used in dry or liquid form. Sprinkle it dry over popcorn.
Corn meal	Muffins, quiche, cornbread and coating for fish, pork and poultry.	
Syrups - Sugar free	Flavor hot cereals, top pancakes, waffles, French toast, breakfast rice cakes and flavor pumpkin porridge.	Sometimes found in the "Diet" section of the grocery store. Available in many flavors. Use in moderation.
Tapioca	Thickener in desserts.	
Whole wheat pancake mix	Pancakes and waffles.	
Wine vinegar	Marinades and salad dressings.	
Wondra	Gravy and soup thickening agent.	This is made with barley making it very healthy.

Never Say Never

Many of you will look at this comprehensive list and think that it was taken from your current shopping list. Living a healthy eating lifestyle does not mean deprivation. It does not mean you can never again eat those delicious foods you enjoy so much. It means making smart decisions at least 95% of the time. When you do choose to have those foods you won't normally be eating in your new lifestyle, consume them in moderation and with very little frequency. It is not detrimental to eat foods high in fat and sugars as long as it is only once in a while.

If you have been eating lean and exercising regularly, occasionally treat yourself to something you really enjoy. Cheese and crackers with a glass of wine, a small bowl of frozen yogurt or ice cream, a peanut butter sandwich or simply a handful of your favorite chips are acceptable in moderation. Allow this for yourself just a couple of times a month, no more than once a week.

Following is a list of foods and beverages you should, more often than not, avoid altogether. It would be best to not even have most of these items in your home. *If it's not there, you can't eat it.* You will notice that some of these items can be found in "fat free" versions, such as the dairy products and mayonnaise, which may be eaten on a daily basis. Dessert items that are available "fat free" contain extremely high amounts of refined sugars and should not be eaten very often. Canned soups and processed lunch meats are much too high in sodium and should also only be eaten in moderation.

Alcoholic beverages
Avocado
Bacon
Beef *

Molasses
Nuts/nut butters (peanut butter)
Oil - animal and vegetable
Olives

Butter
Buttermilk
Caffeinated coffee and tea
Cake
Candy
Cheeses (made with whole milk)
Chocolate
Cookies
Cream
Croissants
Doughnuts
Egg yolks
Frozen yogurt
Fructose
Half-n-half
Honey
Lunch meats - processed
Ice cream
Margarine
Mayonnaise
Milk - whole or 2 %

Pastries
Pie
Salad dressings: Thousand
   Island, Caesar, Bleu Cheese,
   Italian, Ranch, French, Bacon
Salami
Salt - added
Sausage
Seafood ** - Carp, catfish, eel,
   herring, mackerel, salmon
   shark, swordfish and trout.
Shellfish ***
Shortening
Soda pop - soft drinks
Soups - creamed, canned and
   prepackaged
Sour cream
Soybean products
Sugar - table white, brown
Sunflower seeds (roasted or raw)
Tartar Sauce
Whipped cream

* Most cuts are too high in fat. When you do choose to eat beef, select rounds and loins, they are the leanest cuts of beef.
** These fish contain more than 3 grams of fat per three ounce serving.
*** Shellfish contain high levels of cholesterol.

Making Better Decisions

Deciding to eat leaner and healthier is a choice that will forever affect your lifestyle in many positive ways. It is the type of lifestyle, however, that will cause you to consistently make decisions about the food you eat whether it be purchased at the grocery store, prepared at home or ordering food at a restaurant. This chapter is designed to help you make smarter choices by providing answers to those alternative choices.

To begin with, you will read about learning to make decisions you are not yet accustomed to making and selecting foods you are not yet accustomed to eating. *Food Substitutes, Baking Hints*, and *Preparation Alternatives* offer helpful tips on modifying recipes in order to successfully prepare a leaner, healthier meal.

Nowadays, with people being so busy, many meals are eaten at a variety of restaurants, from small cafes, fast food restaurants and street stands to elegant eating establishments. You may find that eating lean can put many limitations on where you choose to dine out. With some knowledge and creativity you will be successful in continuing your lean, healthy eating lifestyle wherever you choose to enjoy your meals. Since for most people eating out occurs more often than eating meals at home, two sections have been designated to helping you become successful in these situations. *Restaurant Food Choices* and *Taboo on the Menu* will show you how to order meals in order to accommodate your lifestyle of eating lean.

Food Substitutes

INSTEAD OF...	TRY...

Dairy:

    Whole or low fat milk — Skim milk, you'll get used to it. If you must, wean yourself from whole milk to 2%, to 1% then to nonfat.

    Creams or half and half — Undiluted, evaporated skimmed milk.

    Sour cream — Nonfat sour cream (mix with a small amount of nonfat milk for better texture and taste).

    Cheese: Hard, cream, cottage — Nonfat cheeses.

    Eggs — Egg whites or egg-product substitutes.

Breads:

    White breads — 100 % whole wheat or stone ground whole wheat; **not** enriched whole wheat bread.

Meats:

    Ground beef — Ground turkey breast.

    Marbled meats (beef & pork) — Lean rounds and loins; eye of round, round tip, top loin, tenderloin, sirloin and top rounds.

Condiments and Miscellaneous:

    Real mayonnaise — Nonfat mayonnaise. This is a great substitute in dishes that do not need to be cooked or baked.

    Syrup — Make your own fruit syrup, sugar free and fat free (See Fruit Glaze recipe). Use sugar free syrup available in many different flavors.

    Salt — Salt free blends are made in an array of flavors to season fish, poultry, vegetables, Italian and Mexican dishes.

INSTEAD OF...	TRY...
Fats:	
Butter or margarine	Omit completely from household. Use non-stick vegetable sprays for pan frying. Fruit spreads, fresh fruits or applesauce to top toast, pancakes, waffles, French toast and the like. There are many butter flavored seasonings on the market that can be sprinkled on potatoes, pasta, vegetables or popcorn. *Butter Buds* can be made into liquid form and used as well on baked potatoes, corn on the cob or in mashed potatoes and vegetables.
Vegetable oils and shortenings	Omit from household, except for non-stick vegetable spray. Water or broths can be used for sautéing along with non-stick vegetable spray. When making marinades replace oil with water or broth.
Snacks:	
Chips and crackers	There are now several "no oil" or "baked" potato and corn (tortilla) chip products on the market. Pretzels and popcorn are also good alternatives. Choose salt-free or low sodium snacks whenever possible. Sometimes you can find bagel chips fat free. Melba toast crackers are low in fat and salt.
Ice Cream	Ice milk, made with nonfat milk. 100% Fruit juice popsicles and fruit sorbets made with no added sugar.
Candy	Seasonal fresh fruit. Try a Fuji apple you won't be disappointed. Raisins, sweet grapes, bananas, oranges, melons in season.
Cakes, cookies and pies	Try recipes in dessert section; cobbler, cookies and muffins.

Preparation Alternatives

When preparing...	Be sure to...
Rice, pre-packaged seasoned	Omit butter or margarine. These rice dishes are seasoned enough to just use water in cooking.
Brown rice, packaged plain	Broth can be used to prepare this rice, or use water if you plan to use rice for rice pancakes.
Marinades, seasoning packets and salad dressings	Omit butter, margarine and oils. If the directions call for oil, use equal amount of water or broth instead. Buy salad dressing mixes that do not require adding oils, butters or margarine.
Pancakes and waffles	Use the same batter to make waffles as you do pancakes. Waffle batter often calls for oil, but it is not necessary.
Egg dishes	Use egg whites only or appropriate amounts of egg substitute (see container for exact amounts).
Sautéing	Use non-stick vegetable spray and broths to prevent sticking.
Salt	Use salt-free blends to flavor your food. Do not add salt, even if the recipe calls for salt. Do not salt your food with table salt. Omit salt from household completely.

Baking Hints

When a recipe calls for...	Use this instead...
Oil, shortening, butter or margarine	Use equivalent amount of unsweetened applesauce.
Whole eggs	Two egg whites for every whole egg. Egg substitutes are also available with no fat and cholesterol that are quite good. Read label for equivalents. I prefer real eggs.
Sugar, white or brown	Cut sugar amounts in half or use dry artificial sweeteners, read labels for equivalents.
Honey or other liquid sweetening agents	Equal amount of fruit juice concentrate.
Fruit glazes prepared with sugar	Make fruit glaze with fruit juice concentrate (See Fruit Glaze recipe).
White flour	100% Whole wheat flour.
Salt	Omit salt from baking.

Restaurant Food Choices

Many restaurants are happy to accommodate special orders making it easier to eat lean while dining out. Always ask your server which low fat or nonfat choices are available if not already noted on the menu. Not all restaurants are going to be willing to specially prepare foods. You may have to try different establishments until you find those willing to accommodate. The following suggestions will be helpful in most restaurants. There are more and more restaurants that are specializing in healthy cooking, look for these types of restaurants in your area.

WHEN ORDERING...	CHOOSE...
Breakfast	
Egg Dishes: Omelettes, scrambled	Order with egg whites only, adding extra egg whites if desired, or ask for an egg substitute. Omit any cheese and sour cream, unless they are available in nonfat. Use vegetable fillings and ham. No sausage, avocado, cream and butter-based sauces such as hollandaise and béarnaise.
Eggs Benedict	To eat this dish leanly, ask for an egg substitute or egg whites scrambled and omit the hollandaise sauce. Ask for the English muffin to be dry; unbuttered.
	Note: If egg substitutes are not available and the cook will not accommodate the "egg whites only" request, order the eggs over-easy and just eat the egg whites.
Potatoes:	Country potatoes with no added fat. Ask that the potatoes you choose be cooked in as little added fat as possible.
Breads: Toast or English muffin	Order your toast "dry" (meaning, without butter). Ask for fruit spreads or jams and jellies and spread on sparingly. Order whole wheat or multi-grain breads.
Bagels	Water-made bagels are lower in fat than bagels made from eggs.

WHEN ORDERING... CHOOSE...

Breakfast (Continued)

French toast	Omit butter and powdered sugar. Use fruit spread, sugar free syrup, applesauce, jams, jellies, cinnamon, fresh fruit or eat them plain. Ask that the French toast be made with whole wheat bread.
Pancakes and waffles	Omit butter. Use fruit spreads, sugar free syrup, applesauce, jams, jellies, fresh fruit, or eat them plain.
Cereal: Cold	Choose the healthiest whole grain cereal available with 1% or skim milk. A small side of fruit can be ordered to top cereal; raisins, banana, berries, peaches. Or sweeten with artificial sweeteners.
Hot	Oatmeal, forina, multi-grain and fat free granola. Omit butter and brown sugar and use 1% or skim milk. To sweeten use sugar free syrup or artificial sweeteners. A small side of fresh fruit can be ordered to top cereal; raisins, banana, berries, peaches.
Breakfast meat:	Ham slices are your best choice. Bacon and sausage are not an option. Steak usually isn't that lean in a restaurant.

Lunch

Salad: Green	Ask for the dressing to be served "on the side" so you control how much is poured on your salad. Ask for fat free or lowfat dressings, if not available use your favorite dressing in moderation. You can always have no dressing at all. Omit cheese, sunflower seeds, nuts, egg yolks, olives and avocado. Be sure not to over do it on the croutons and salad dressing. Romaine, red leaf lettuce or spinach are nutritionally preferred over ice-berg (head) lettuce.

WHEN ORDERING...   CHOOSE...

Lunch(Continued)

Salad (Continued):

Coleslaw, potato and pasta. — Only if made with nonfat mayonnaise and no oil. Some potato and pasta salads include egg yolks which you do not want.

Fruit — No marshmallow cream, whipping cream, whipped topping or added sugar. Order fresh fruit salad in fruits own juice.

Soups: — Broth soups are preferable; vegetable, turkey, chicken, barley or minestrone. Beef used in soups is usually not very lean and definitely stay away from cream soups. Keep it light on the crackers. Sorry, no white clam chowder.

Bread as a side dish: — Whole wheat or multi-grain if available. Order without butter or olive oil.

Bread for sandwiches: — Whole wheat or multi-grain. Order "light" or low calorie bread when available.

Sandwiches: — No grilled sandwiches. No mayonnaise, mayonnaise dressings, mayonnaise based sauces, cheeses or cream cheese, unless they are available in nonfat. No avocado, pastrami, corned beef, bologna, sausage, liverwurst, salami, bacon or mortadella. No egg, tuna, chicken, or turkey salad sandwiches, much too much fat. Acceptable ingredients: Mustard, lettuce, tomato, pickles, chili peppers, spouts, bell peppers, onions, mushrooms. Stick with white turkey or chicken meat, roast beef, lean ham and vegetable sandwiches (except avocados).

Burgers: — Skinless chicken breast, lean ground turkey and most garden burgers are acceptable. No cheese, avocado, bacon, mayonnaise or mayonnaise based sauces or grilled

WHEN ORDERING...   *CHOOSE...*

Lunch(Continued)

Burgers (Continued):

onions. Acceptable ingredients: Mustard, lettuce, tomato, pickles, relish, chili peppers, spouts, bell peppers, fresh onions and mushrooms.

Chips: Fat free pretzels, no-oil (baked) tortilla chips, plain bagel chips; all preferably salt-free.

Chicken entrees: See suggestions listed under "Dinner".

Fish entrees: See suggestions listed under "Dinner".

Dinner

Salad and soup: See suggestions listed under "Lunch".

Bread as a side dish: Whole wheat or multi-grain when available. Don't butter bread or dip in olive oil. No cheese or garlic bread. Ask for bread plain and warmed, if desired.

Main course:

  Meats

Grilled or broiled. If barbecued, no extra sauce. No heavy cream or butter sauces. Most chutney or salsa toppings, are acceptable, ask for them to be served "on the side".

  Poultry:
  Chicken and Turkey

White meat only. Have skin removed or remove it yourself. Grilled, baked, broiled or barbecued. If barbecued, no extra sauce. No heavy cream or butter sauces. Most chutney or salsa toppings are acceptable, ask for them to be served "on the side". Check ingredients for added fat whenever possible.

  Duck

Do not order. Duck is too high in fat.

WHEN ORDERING... CHOOSE...

Dinner (Continued)

Main Course (Continued):

Fish — Grilled, broiled, baked, barbecued, poached or steamed. No heavy cream or butter sauces. No tartar sauce, unless fat free. Most chutney or salsa toppings are acceptable, ask for them to be served "on the side". Check ingredients for added fat whenever possible.

Potato:

Baked — Ask for a "dry" baked potato (served without butter). Topping options sometimes include green onions, chives, nonfat sour cream, salsa.

Other potatoes: Red, white, mashed, scalloped, fried. — Mashed potatoes are not usually made very lean in restaurants. If you order them omit the gravy and butter. Do not order scalloped potatoes or French fries. Often small red or white potatoes are served as a side dish. Ask for them with no added fat such as with olive oil, vegetable oil, fried or buttered. Steamed or baked is best.

Rice: Order brown or brown with wild rice together when available. Rice pilaf is usually made with white rice which is not as nutritious as brown rice.

Pasta: Plain, with steamed vegetables or with a fresh tomato sauce. Most marinaras are made with olive oil, order "light" on the sauce. No heavy cream or butter sauces. Pasta with grilled chicken breast or fish and vegetables, with no sauce may be an option.

Vegetables: Steamed to your liking; crisp to well-done.

Dessert: Fresh fruit, fruit sorbets. Ask if there are any healthy dessert choices.

Taboo on the Menu

A word or two can mean a thousand calories and a few inches of fat added to your stomach and thighs. Not all dishes on the menu are explained in detail, leaving the surprise to appear when you are served. This list of menu items will steer you away from those dishes that are prepared with high levels of fat and sugars. Items listed below are found on menus of varying restaurants. Very few dessert dishes are mentioned, as there are very few desserts available in restaurants, made with small amounts of fat and sugar. Also not listed, are dishes prepared with obviously large amounts of cheese or dishes containing sausage as a main ingredient, these should be out of the question.

à la king - Food that is diced and prepared in a rich cream sauce.
à la mode - Topped with vanilla ice cream.
Albert sauce - Horseradish sauce with a flour, cream and butter base.
allemande sauce - This sauce is thickened with egg yolks (a.k.a. **parisienne sauce**).
allumettes - Hors d'oeuvres made with puff pastry usually filled with flavored butters, cheeses or sweeter dessert fillings. Allumettes are also named for thinly cut fried potatoes.
amandine or almondine - Dishes that are generously garnished with almonds.
andalouse sauce - Mayonnaise based sauce.
angels on horseback - Bacon-wrapped oysters served on buttered toast. The hot and spicy version of this hors d'oeuvre is known as **"devils on horseback."**
anglaise - Food that has been prepared by coating with bread crumbs then frying.
antipasto - Meaning "before the pasta". A plate of hors d'oeuvres usually including cheese, olives, smoked meats or salamis and marinated vegetables.
au gratin - A topping that is broiled to golden brown, made up of bread crumbs and butter or grated cheese.

béarnaise sauce - Sauce containing egg yolks, butter, wine, vinegar, shallots and tarragon. Served with fish, eggs, meats and vegetables.
béchamel sauce - Sauce made with butter, milk and flour.
beurre - This word means "butter" in French, "au beurre" means cooked in butter.
bisque - Soup that has a cream base used for making it rich and thick.
bouchée - A puff pastry shell sometimes filled with creamed seafood.
brandade - Puree containing olive oil, milk, cream, garlic and a salted or smoked fish.
buñuelo - A Mexican pastry deep-fried and sprinkled with cinnamon and sugar.

carbonara - Pasta smothered with a rich cream sauce made up of eggs, cream, Parmesan cheese and bacon bits.

chalupa - Corn tortilla dough formed into the shape of a small boat, deep-fried and filled with cheese, shredded meat and vegetables, or any combination thereof.

chicken Kiev - Boned chicken breast that is prepared by shaping the meat around a chunk of butter, sometimes herbed butter, then dipped in egg, coated with bread crumbs and deep fried until done.

chicken Tetrazzini - Pasta and chicken pieces covered with a creamy cheese sauce. Sometimes turkey is used, hence, **turkey Tetrazzini**.

chiles rellenos - Green chiles that are stuffed with cheese, covered with egg batter and deep-fried.

chimichanga - Deep-fried burrito usually topped with guacamole, cheese and sour cream.

coquilles St. Jacques - Scallops bathing in a rich cream wine sauce topped with cheese or bread crumbs.

cordon bleu - Chicken and veal are most commonly used in this dish, as well as thin slices of ham and Swiss or Gruyere cheese. The meats and cheese are alternately stacked then breaded and sautéed until done.

croissant - A roll that is very buttery and flaky. Can be eaten as a dessert or breakfast pastry, a sandwich bread or accompaniment at any meal.

croquette - Minced meat or vegetables blended with a rich white sauce formed into bite-sized pieces, coated with bread crumbs then deep-fried.

dauphine - These are a potato croquette. Combining a puff pastry dough with mashed or pureed potatoes, forming into bite-sized balls, rolled in bread crumbs and deep-fried.

deep-fry - Don't even think about it! Foods cooked in very hot oil or lard.

eggs Benedict - English muffin halves topped with ham or Canadian bacon, a poached egg and hollandaise sauce.

fish - A few of the popular fish high in fat include salmon, rainbow trout, mackerel, Atlantic herring, yellowtail and shad. Moderately-fat fish that are between 2 1/2 % and 6% fat include, shark, swordfish, tuna, striped bass, bluefish and barracuda. Lean fish which contain up to 2 1/2% fat are halibut, flounder, red snapper, rockfish, black sea bass, sturgeon, cod, brook trout, haddock, and ocean perch.

flauta - Corn tortilla rolled and stuffed with chicken, pork or beef then fried until golden brown.

focaccia - A delicious Italian bread that is generously coated with olive oil and topped with herbs.

fritto - Italian for food that is dipped in batter then deep-fried.

fry bread - Also known as Indian fry bread. Bread that has been deep-fried and usually served hot, sometimes smothered in cinnamon-sugar.

German potato salad - Not the leanest of potato salads, commonly made with bacon, bacon fat drippings and sugar.
goulash - This dish is like a stew served over buttery noodles and topped with sour cream.
guacamole - A Mexican side dish or dip. Main ingredient is mashed avocados seasoned with lemon juice and sometimes salsa, green onions and cilantro.

hollandaise sauce - A rich and creamy sauce made with egg yolks, butter and lemon juice.

meunière - A style of preparing food that consists of a light dusting of flour then sautéing in butter until done.
milanaise - Pasta smothered in butter and cheese then topped with tomato sauce, ham, mushrooms, tongue and truffles.
Milanese - Food that is dipped in an egg batter, coated with a bread crumb and cheese mixture then fried in butter.
Mornay sauce - A sauce with a milk, butter and flour base. Cheese and any combination of egg yolks, cream and broth is then added to make the sauce richer and creamier.
mousseline sauce - Hollandaise sauce that has added whipped cream or egg whites to make the sauce lighter in consistency.

Nantua sauce - A sauce made with milk, butter, flour, cream and crayfish butter. Often served with seafood and egg dishes.
Newburg - Something made "Newburg" contains a rich sauce made with egg yolks, butter, cream and sherry.
normande sauce - This sauce has a fish-stock base with added butter, egg yolks and cream.

parisienne sauce - See **allemande sauce.**
parmigiana - Food that is prepared by being dipped in egg batter, coated with bread crumbs and topped with generous amounts of Parmesan cheese, then sautéed. Tomato sauce is then poured over the top just before serving. Sometimes mozzarella cheese is added.
pesto - Known as the "green sauce", pesto is most often served on pasta. It is made by pureeing together fresh basil leaves, olive oil, garlic, pine nuts and Parmesan cheese. The French call this sauce **pistou**. (Also as known by the French, pistou is a soup that is similar to minestrone but flavored with basil and garlic.)

quesadilla - Flour or corn tortillas that sandwich cheese with or without any combination of shredded meat, refried beans, onions and salsa. The tortilla is broiled or fried in a hot pan until middle is melted and tortillas are slightly browned.

queso - Spanish word meaning "cheese".

quiche - Real men don't eat quiche and neither should you (unless you make the quiche recipe in *Eat to be Lean*). A light, flaky pastry shell filled with a combination of mostly cheese, eggs and cream. Other ingredients such as onions, mushrooms, bacon, spinach and sausage are used to further flavor the dish.

ratatouille - A combination of vegetables that are cooked by simmering in olive oil.

rémoulade - A cold sauce made with mayonnaise, mustard, anchovies, capers, gherkins, herbs and seasonings.

sauté - Preparing foods by means of quickly cooking in hot oil or butter in a skillet over high heat.

scaloppini - Thin scallops of meat coated in flour then sautéed in butter and/or olive oil, then covered with a sauce of wine, tomatoes or mushrooms.

schnitzel - Meat dipped in an egg batter, coated with a breading then fried to doneness.

soubise - Another delicious white creamy sauce made with butter, milk, flour, cream and pureed cook onions.

soufflé - A dish in which the main ingredient is egg yolks. Cheese, meat, vegetables and seafood are added to flavor.

tartar sauce - A mayonnaise based sauce blended with minced dill pickles, shallots and sometimes capers.

tempura - Bite-sized pieces of meats, poultry, seafood and vegetables

Lattes, Mochas, Breves & More

So you just can't do without that daily espresso drink? Well, until you decide to kick the habit and save yourself numerous extra calories, not to mention the amount of money you could be saving and putting towards a gym membership, here are some alternatives to that cup of Java.

Living in the greater Seattle area has its advantages when it comes to espresso drinks. There is virtually an espresso stand or coffee cafe within a block or two of everywhere. Because of the fierce competition, many espresso stands are accommodating the needs of those who choose not to go all out with the whole milk, flavored syrups, whipping cream and various toppings, making it very convenient to find a low-calorie, low sugar, great tasting espresso drink.

Though most people drink espressos for the caffeine "buzz" and terrific flavors, there are those who just enjoy the flavor of the coffee and any added flavorings. Fortunately for these people, ordering a decaf espresso would be an inconsequential change, and a much wiser choice. I recommend you start weaning yourself away from caffeine as soon as possible. Some side effects caused by caffeine include hypertension (high blood pressure), ulcers, hypoglycemia, artery disorders, heart aggravations, insomnia, hypothyroidism, heartburn and more. Whether you order your coffee drinks out or make them at home, start by blending half decaf and half regular coffee together. Every couple of weeks increase the ratio of decaffeinated coffee until you are drinking strictly decaf. This can be accomplished with whole bean or canned coffees. Whole bean coffee has a tremendous amount of body and flavor which is not lost in the process of eliminating the caffeine. Using ground, decaffeinated, whole bean coffee may be more pleasing to your taste buds when phasing out caffeine. Staying away from caffeine includes eliminating tea, which is known to have more caffeine than coffee, and chocolate. Decaffeinated herbal teas are a good substitute and also come in a variety of flavors.

Listed are the most commonly ordered coffee drinks and their traditional ingredients. Shown next to that is an alternative way to order each drink. Moderation should always be exercised in regard to frequency and size of drinks. If you make these drinks at home it is convenient to have on hand the necessary ingredients to make a low-to-no fat, sugar-free espresso drinks. If you normally buy your coffee drinks away from home, you may have to try a few different espresso stands or coffee cafes until you find one that will be accommodating.

There are a few important factors to keep in mind when making or ordering your espresso drinks; decaf, nonfat, sugar free and eight ounce. This may seem boring compared to what you are used to ordering, and a great way to ruin a perfectly tasty cup of Java, but your health should take priority. It may take a few drinks to become accustom to the new changes. If need be, begin by changing one ingredient at a time, for instance, order your espresso drinks with half decaf, half regular coffee. Next, go from whole milk to 2%, to 1%, eventually ordering them with nonfat milk. After you get used to that, try a sugar-free, flavored syrup. If this whole idea seems simply unbearable, then make that double tall, whole milk mocha with hazelnut flavoring, whipped cream and chocolate topping a monthly treat instead of a daily indulgence.

TRADITIONAL   *ALTERNATIVE*

Espresso:
Espresso

Espresso:
Decaf espresso

Cappuccino:
Espresso
Foamed milk

Cappuccino:
Decaf espresso
Foamed nonfat milk

Latteccino:
Espresso
Steamed milk
Foamed milk

Latteccino:
Decaf espresso
Steamed nonfat milk
Foamed nonfat milk

Latte:
Espresso
Steamed milk
Dollop of foam

Latte:
Decaf espresso
Steamed nonfat milk
Dollop of foam

TRADITIONAL	ALTERNATIVE
Flavored Latte: Espresso Steamed milk Flavored syrup Dollop of foam	**Flavored Latte:** Decaf Espresso Steamed nonfat milk Flavored sugar-free syrup Dollop of foam

Mocha:
Espresso
Steamed milk
Creme de Cacao
   or
Chocolate syrup
Whipping cream
Powdered sweet chocolate
   or
Chocolate sprinkles
	Mocha:
	Decaf espresso
	Steamed nonfat milk
	Sugar-free Creme de Cacao
	   or
	Sugar/fat free chocolate mix
	NO whipping cream
	NO topping

Breve: Espresso Steamed Cream	**Breve:** Don't even think about it, order a cafe royal instead
Cafe Royal: Espresso Steamed condensed milk	**Cafe Royal:** Decaf espresso Steamed condensed nonfat milk

Flavored Mocha:
Espresso
Steamed milk
Creme de Cacao
   or
Chocolate syrup
Flavored syrup
Whipping cream
Powdered sweet chocolate
   or
Chocolate sprinkles
	Flavored Mocha:
	Decaf espresso
	Steamed nonfat milk
	Sugar-free Creme de Cacao
	   or
	Sugar/fat free chocolate mix
	Flavored sugar-free syrup
	NO whipping cream
	NO topping

There are many ways to order these drinks in regard to quantity of ingredients. Cup sizes range from eight ounces all the way up to a 20 ounce size (espresso comes in small 1-2 ounce demitasse). Some coffee stands may offer even larger sizes. The number of shots of espresso normally range from one to four, with each shot equalling one ounce. Stick to the eight ounce size with one shot of espresso to keep the calories down.

Also popular are the "iced" espresso drinks that are very refreshing during the hot summer months. The espresso is chilled then poured over ice along with the milk and any added flavorings. No foam accompanies these drinks. Granitas are drinks made in a special machine blending finely granulated ice, flavorings and sometimes half and half, creating a slush-like drink. Coffee and fruit flavorings are the most common. Since these drinks are pre-made, it is not likely you will be able to find them low calorie and sugar-free.

There may be slight variations in the way the drinks are made depending on who makes them. Many establishments develop their own concoctions using special chocolates, yogurt, food coloring, eggnog, pumpkin and fruit. The competition among espresso stand owners keeps the variety of drinks ever changing. Be sure to check the ingredients before you order if you are unsure.

So You Need to Gain a Few Pounds?

Are you one of the few thin people on this planet who, no matter what you do, cannot seem to gain an ounce of weight, and keep it on? Since a majority of this nation's weight problem is losing weight, very little attention has been paid to those at the other end of the spectrum. Gaining weight, and keeping it on, is just as much a frustrating struggle as it is to lose weight and keep it off.

My best advice in two words is "eat" and "exercise". The ability to put on lean body mass depends greatly on the amount of food you eat and the amount of weight training you do. You must eat, eat, and eat some more, your body needs the calories. You need protein for muscle and tissue growth and carbohydrates for energy. Usually thin people can afford to eat a few more fat calories but should not go overboard. You want the body mass you put on to be lean, not fat. You also want to keep those arteries clean and free of fat and cholesterol build-up. If you think you already eat a lot, eat more! Do not go more than three hours without food. Pack food in a small tote cooler and keep it near so you always have access to healthy food. Try the recipe at the end of this chapter as a snack. It is an easy to prepare shake loaded with calories high in protein and carbohydrates. It has no fat and tastes great. I wish I could drink them, but extra calories are not something my body needs.

Exercising with weights is another effective way to put on lean muscle mass and strength. You must be sure to eat enough food for muscle growth and to make up for the extra calories you will be utilizing during exercise. Keep your aerobic exercise minimal, 2-3 times per week no more than twenty minutes at a time. If you are not already participating in an exercise program, be sure to start slow for the first couple of months, performing sets of 10-15 repetitions. Eventually, you will work yourself into doing sets of 6-8 repetitions with heavier weights to help increase your muscle mass.

Eating more and weight training are your two biggest tools for gaining lean muscle mass. You must eat the right foods for optimum results. The foods suggested in *Eat to be Lean* are the types of foods you should be eating. Indulge in quantity and frequency of meals. You will no doubt get tired of eating and preparing your daily meals but it's what has to be done in order to obtain your goals.

Weight Gain Shake

1 - 12 oz. Can evaporated skimmed milk
1/2 Cup nonfat dry milk powder
1 Banana
1 Cup frozen fruit, unsweetened (strawberries, peaches, berries)
1 Cup unsweetened fruit juice (make juice with less water than required for higher calorie content)

Place all ingredients in blender and blend until smooth. Put canned milk in the refrigerator to ensure drinks will be cool and refreshing. Try adding a container of yogurt or some pumpkin for extra calories and flavor. Each drink, as prepared above, contains approximately 600 calories. Enjoy!!

Exercise

Eat to be Lean would not be complete without a discussion about exercise. Don't let the word "exercise" intimidate you. Simply stated it means "body movement". You must keep your body moving to keep blood flowing for good circulation and keep muscles moving to prevent atrophy. You must also challenge your muscles to increase strength and prevent or reverse osteoporosis, and challenge your heart to keep it strong and healthy.

In order to achieve your goals of good health and appearance you **must** incorporate good nutrition and eating lean, aerobic exercise and resistive weight training into your daily life. There is no possible way to reach your goals by combining only one or two of these aspects. Your lifestyle must include all of them, simultaneously, in order to succeed. Otherwise, you will be fighting a loosing battle. I have personally been there and continue to observe this type of dead-end behavior in the gym I co-own and in other gyms and health club facilities where I have personally trained. People are putting forth great effort toward their workout routine only to go home and negate everything they have accomplished by eating all the wrong foods, or all the right foods, in the wrong quantities. On the other hand, there are people who eat right but don't exercise and wonder why they still have too much body fat or no strength and muscle tone. You have to participate and incorporate the whole package to receive optimal results. *Your results are directly dependent on your efforts.*

Aerobic exercise is necessary to utilize, or burn off, the excess fat your body has stored and to help keep it off. Eating lean will also help prevent excess storage of body fat. Aerobic exercise is performed by exercising large muscle groups, for long durations of time (20-60 consecutive minutes), keeping your heartbeats per minute in aerobic range - 55% - 85% of your maximum heart rate. To calculate your aerobic heart rate subtract your age from 220 (maximum heart rate). Multiply that number by .55 and .85. This will give you your aerobic heart range in beats per minute.

Maximum heart rate	=	220		
Less your age	-	40		
		180		180
Multiply 55% - 85%	x	.55		.85
Aerobic Heart Rate	=	**99**	-	**153**
(Beats per minute)				
15 Second Count	=	25	-	38

Cycling, running/jogging, rowing, aerobic classes, brisk walking, roller skating, stair climbing and swimming are common forms of aerobic exercise. This should be done at least three times per week. Aerobic exercise also increases your metabolism and strengthens your heart and lungs.

Weight training exercises should be performed no less than two times a week, for a presently sedentary person, and 3-5 days a week for the most benefit. Weight training increases muscle and joint strength, increases bone density and increases basal metabolic rate - resting metabolism. Lean body mass (muscle) uses more calories per day to maintain than body fat, that is why your metabolism increases the more muscle you have.

The benefits of exercise are abundant. There are so many enjoyable activities that exercise not only your body, but your mind and soul as well. Bicycle riding, swimming, brisk walking, roller skating, hiking, weight lifting, basketball and dance are to name just a few. Higher energy levels, greater self-confidence and self-esteem, better health and a higher quality of life are common benefits achieved through regular exercise. Exercise is not discriminatory, virtually everyone can perform some form of exercise even if it is from a chair or their bed. Start exercising today, get yourself and your family involved. Ask a friend to join you. If I could have things my way, everybody would be exercising and feeling terrific.

Menu Ideas

Breakfast/Brunch Ideas

French Toast
Rice pancakes
Ham and egg on toast
Bagel with fruit or nonfat cream cheese

Pancakes
Waffles
Muffins with milk or juice
Whole wheat toast or low fat biscuits

Egg Dishes

Omelette or scrambles eggs whites with any of the following:

Onions	Mushrooms
Bell peppers	Celery
Tomatoes	Salsa
Potato	Ham
Zucchini	Ground turkey burger
Broccoli	Steak slices
Spinach	Canadian bacon

Omelette fillings:
- Chili/chili casserole
- Spaghetti sauce
- Vegetables
- Ham
- Manicotti filling
- Stuffed bell pepper mixture

Egg Hash:
- Diced potatoes
- Onions
- Celery
- Ground turkey burger
- Bell peppers
- Barbecue sauce

Breakfast tostada
Breakfast burritos
Quiche

Toppings for egg dishes: Nonfat sour cream, nonfat cheese, salsa, marinara, sliced/diced bell peppers, onions, tomatoes, and green chilies.

Potatoes

Fried mashed potatoes (a real favorite here!).
Microwave potatoes diced or sliced and fried.
Hash browns or shredded potatoes, frozen or fresh.

Variations: Add chopped onions, bell peppers, garlic.

Breakfast Meats

Lean ham
Steaks, small lean cut eye of round
Smoked turkey breast
Canadian bacon

Cereal

Cold cereal with nonfat milk and fruit: raisins, bananas, peaches, berries.

Hot cereal with nonfat milk and fruits, as listed above, applesauce or sugar free syrup.

Pumpkin porridge.

Lunch Ideas

Sandwiches

Cold	Hot
Sliced steak *	Barbecue beef *
Fried egg with or without ham/Canadian bacon slices	Barbecue pork *
Tuna salad	Philly-style steak sandwich *
Tuna/egg salad	French dip *
Chicken or turkey salad *	
Egg salad	

Cold or Hot
Barbecue chicken breasts   Meatloaf *

Bowl of...(with cornbread or whole wheat rolls)

Turkey chili
Clam chowder
Vegetable beef soup

Chicken or turkey soup (many variations)
Chili casserole

Other ideas

Burritos
Spaghetti
Mini pizza

Lasagna
Spaghetti sauce or chili over mashed or diced potatoes

* Made from leftovers.

Side dishes and/or other accompaniments

Fruit or fruit salad
No-oil (baked) chips and salsa
Canned beans

Pasta salad
Green salad

Dinner Ideas

These ideas do not include the side dishes (i.e., pasta, potatoes, rice, salads, vegetables, etc., see Side Dishes)

Chicken Breast

Chicken stroganoff
Sautéed in marinara
Breaded/coated and baked

Barbecued
Kebabs
Pan-fried

Turkey Breast (whole or ground)

Crock pot cooked with gravy
Meatloaf or meatballs
Turkey Chili with Cornbread

Turkey burgers with French fries
Turkey stroganoff

Beef

Stew
Boneless spareribs baked, barbecued or cooked in crock pot
Kebabs

Crock pot Eye of Round, with gravy
London broil, broiled or barbecued
Beef stroganoff

Pork

Pork Loin roast or chops cooked in crock pot, with gravy
Pork chops coated and baked

Boneless spareribs baked, barbecued or cooked in crock pot with gravy

Fish

Orange Roughy/Petrale Sole/Sole/Snapper - Coated and baked, steamed, pan fried, poached or seasoned and baked.
Swordfish/Halibut/Shark - Barbecued, broiled, kebabs.

Mexican dishes

- Burritos
- Chili casserole
- Tostada
- Soft tacos
- Quesadillas
- Fajitas

Italian and pasta dishes

- Spaghetti sauce over pasta
- Lasagna
- Stuffed pasta shells
- Manicotti
- Pizza

Vegetable dishes

- Stuffed bell peppers
- Stuffed cabbage rolls

Side Dishes

Potato

- Mashed potatoes
- Baked potato, plain or baked potato splurge
- Twice baked or stuffed
- Sliced, seasoned fries
- Diced with peppers, onions, garlic
- Potato skins
- French fries

Pasta

- Pasta primavera with angel hair pasta
- Cous cous

Rice (brown or wild)

- Rice cooked with broth or water, with added chopped green onions and water chestnuts.
- Seasoned rice, prepackaged
- Veggie rice cakes

Stuffing/dressing

- With added mushrooms, onions, celery

Salads

Green leaf
Coleslaw
Potato
Spinach
Fruit

Vegetables

Fresh, steamed
Sauté

Snack or Appetizer Ideas

Popcorn, air-popped sprinkled
   with butter-flavored seasonings
Muffins
Baked corn chips with salsa
   and bean dip
Pretzels
Nonfat yogurt

Quesadillas
Layered bean dip with chips or
   tortillas
Potato skins
Fruits
Nonfat cottage cheese and fruit
100% Fruit juice popsicles

Dessert Ideas

Pumpkin cookies
Strawberry shortcake with cream
   cheese (Any berries can be used)
Fruit sorbet - no sugar added

Fruit salad
100% Fruit juice popsicles
Fruit cobbler (peach, berry, apple)
Muffins

Recipes

Breakfast/Brunch
Muffins
Lunch
Dinner
Side Dishes
Appetizers
Desserts

The kitchen is reorganized, the food inventory depicts a lean and healthy eating lifestyle, now what do you do with it all? The following recipes will show you how to put it all together to create delicious, healthy and easy to prepare meals.

For those of you fond of cooking, the recipes in this section will be quite simple and gratifying. Unfortunately, it seems that most people would rather not cook because they either don't enjoy it, are intimidated by having to follow recipes or simply don't have the time. My goal is to help you become more comfortable and confident with cooking, learning to use recipes as a foundation for creating food dishes. You will also learn time-saving ideas to make preparation more simple.

One of the most difficult tasks an experienced cook faces is putting prepared dishes into recipe form. When you are used to cooking with some of this and a dash of that, exact amounts can be very puzzling. With a lot of patience and measuring I have successfully conquered this task. These recipes were created from everyday, ordinary foods for the typical "meat and potato" appetite. There are no fancy cooking methods with unheard of ingredients or sauces that take days to prepare. Often variations are offered giving you plenty of ideas and options. Quantities can be plentiful or prepared for one.

It is helpful to spend a few minutes planning the week's dinners, keeping lunches in mind. Whenever possible, make large enough quantities to have enough left-overs for future lunches or dinners. If you are serving two, cook for four, if you are serving four, cook enough for six. It takes just a few extra minutes of preparation time to make extras. When I make mashed potatoes, I peel an extra 3-6 potatoes giving me enough left over to have fried mashed potatoes for breakfast and chili over potatoes for lunch. Take a little extra time on the weekends to get ahead by chopping and dicing ingredients you most often use during the week. Since I use a lot of onions and bell peppers, I dice two or three of each and place them in separate airtight containers in the refrigerator for use during the week, this is a great time-saver.

Most of the ingredients are found on the *Master Grocery List* of groceries. The ingredients appearing in bold print, in some recipes, indicate items that are not on the *Master Grocery List*. Read each recipe carefully, noting ingredients you may not have in stock. This enables you to plan ahead and pick this item up on your next trip to the store. Sometimes the ingredient can be optional.

A few of the recipes do not include exact amounts, allowing serving sizes to vary. The purpose of this approach is to teach you that cooking can be made simple and is infinite in its creative possibilities. You will learn that if you don't like a particular ingredient, such as onions, leave them out. If you don't like beans in your chili, leave them out. The creativity lies within your own taste buds. Learn to use recipes as guidelines in your cooking. You are given the basic concept of how to prepare each dish, from there you can add your own personal touches. Most of the time the cooking methods are more important than the ingredients themselves. Relax and enjoy yourself. You will learn that cooking can be fun, fast and easy.

Take time to read through each recipe before you begin. There may be helpful hints and variations to the recipe you choose. Review the *Menu Ideas* to help design your next meal and try to plan ahead. Often what you make for dinner will determine what lunch will be the following day or two. For example, if you make an eye of round roast for dinner, with potatoes, gravy and vegetables, lunches to follow could be barbecue beef sandwiches, beef burritos, tacos or simply heated up leftovers.

It takes time to get used to eating lean. Your taste buds, as well as your cooking habits, need adjustment. Enjoy the creativeness of cooking and the great flavors you can make with healthy foods.

Breakfast/Brunch

Breakfast Favorites:
French Toast
Pancakes and Waffles
Rice Pancakes

Hot Cereals:
Pumpkin Porridge
Oats and Multi-grain Cereals

Egg Dishes:
Toppings for Egg Dishes
Omelettes
Philly-style Steak Omelette
Scrambled Eggs - Fancy
Egg Hash
Breakfast Burritos
Breakfast Tostadas
Easy Quiche

Breakfast Potatoes:
Fried Mashed Potatoes
Hash Browns
Fried Diced Potatoes

Breakfast Favorites

French Toast

Whole wheat bread, sliced
Egg whites (one for each piece of bread)
Dash of cinnamon
1/4 -1/2 tsp. Vanilla

Coat skillet or griddle with non-stick cooking spray, pre-heat over medium heat. In small bowl, with whisk or fork, rapidly beat egg whites, cinnamon and vanilla. Place egg mixture in shallow dish, like a pie plate, something wide enough to fit a whole slice of bread. Place one slice of bread at a time in egg batter, coat on both sides. Put bread slices on heated skillet, be careful not to overlap. Cook over medium heat until brown on both sides. Remove from pan and serve.

Top with: Sugar free syrup, applesauce, fruit spreads, fresh berries or fruit glaze. Warm the toppings in a microwave or on the stove top, just enough to take the chill off. It helps to keep the French toast from getting cold.

Pancakes and Waffles

Whole wheat pancake mix

Make pancake batter according to instructions. Use pancake batter to make waffles as well. Waffle batters normally call for added vegetable oil to prevent sticking to waffle iron. By coating the waffle iron with non-stick cooking spray you can prevent sticking and omit the oil.

Variations: To add a little pizazz to waffles and pancakes try adding any one or more of the following ingredients in small amounts to the batter (approximately 1/4 cup to 1 cup of batter):

- Chopped apple
- Pumpkin
- Unsweetened applesauce
- Pureed bananas
- Raisins
- Rolled oats
- Berries

Top with: Sugar free syrup, applesauce, fruit spreads, fresh berries or fruit glaze. Warm the toppings in a microwave or on the stove top, just enough to take the chill off and keep the pancakes and waffles from getting cold too fast.

Rice-Pancakes

2 Cups cooked brown rice, cooled.
   Leftover rice works well for
   this recipe.
5 Egg whites

1/4 tsp. Cinnamon
1/2 tsp. Vanilla or maple extract
Dash of nutmeg

In medium sized bowl, combine all ingredients, blending with a spoon. Batter should be thick, not soupy. Let stand for 10 minutes. Coat skillet or griddle with non-stick cooking spray, pre-heat over medium heat. Lightly stir batter, pour or spoon batter onto skillet making 4" pancakes. Cook until firm and browned on both sides. Remove from pan and serve. Makes 6-8 pancakes.

Top with: Sugar free syrup, applesauce, fruit spreads, fresh berries or fruit glaze. Warm the toppings in a microwave or on the stove top, just enough to take the chill off. It also helps to keep the rice-pancakes from getting cold too fast.

Note: This recipe can be modified and served as a dinner side dish. See Veggie Rice Cakes in "Side Dish Recipes" section.

Hot-Cereals

Pumpkin Porridge

Great for kids and loaded with vitamins.

Canned pumpkin
Evaporated skimmed milk

Dash of cinnamon and/or nutmeg
or dash or two of **pumpkin pie spice**

Variations: Add in raisins, sugar free maple syrup, sweeteners.

Spoon desired amount of pumpkin into sauce pan. Gradually add milk and stir until desired consistency. Add in raisins or sweeteners and cook over medium heat until warmed thoroughly. This is a great way to get your vitamin "A", and curb any cravings for pumpkin pie.

Oats and Multi-grain Cereals

Oatmeal comes in many variations these days. Instant oatmeal cereals are often high in sugar and sodium, stay away from those. Regular oats can be prepared in the microwave or on the stove top. I prefer old fashioned rolled oats for the texture. If a thicker, pastier oatmeal is desired try the "quick" oats.

Zoom is a cereal made with 100% whole wheat with no added sugars, fats or sodium. This can be mixed with the oatmeal for a different flavor and texture. I prefer to make hot cereals with less water than called for on the instructions for a chewier texture.

Variations: Top hot cereal with nonfat milk or evaporated skimmed milk, stir in raisins, berries, bananas or sugar-free maple syrup. Unsweetened applesauce also makes a flavorful topping. For added flavor add a 1/4 teaspoon of vanilla or maple extract to the cereal as it is cooking or a 1/4 cup of chopped apple. If you like a crunchy texture, top with a tablespoon or two of *Grapenuts*.

Egg Dishes

If making omelettes or scrambled eggs without egg yolks is a change you are not yet willing to make, try omitting half of the yolks, or using an egg product substitute. The following recipes are made with egg whites only. Some revisions may have to be made when using egg substitutes, read carton for instructions. The object is to not use any egg yolks at all in your cooking and baking. Quantities are not that important in the breakfast dishes and using more or less of an ingredient will not ruin the dish. Use the amount of filling and eggs that are adequate for the number of servings you are preparing. Two egg whites are equivalent to one whole egg.

Toppings for Egg Dishes

Nonfat sour cream
Salsa
Sliced/diced onion
Sliced/diced bell pepper

Nonfat cheese
Marinara sauce
Sliced/diced tomatoes
Green chilies, diced

Omelettes

Omelette filling, your choice
See *Breakfast Ideas,* Chapter IX

Egg whites

This may seem vague, but the trick is in the preparation of the omelette shell. To follow is how to prepare a Denver omelette that serves two to three people.

1/4 Cup chopped onions
1/4 Cup chopped bell peppers

1/2 Cup diced, lean ham
8 Egg whites
Dash of **Tabasco sauce** (optional)

Lightly beat egg whites and Tabasco sauce in small bowl; set aside. Coat 10"-12" skillet with non-stick cooking spray, preheat over medium-high heat. Add onions, bell peppers and ham, cook for 8-10 minutes until vegetables are tender and ham is browned, remove from pan and set aside. Spray skillet again with non-stick cooking spray, place over medium heat until pan becomes warmed. Pour in egg whites and cover with a lid. Cook for approximately 7-10 minutes or until eggs are cooked all the way through. Lay filling over half the eggs, as in a half circle. Flip the other side of the eggs over on top of the filling to form an omelette, cut in half or thirds and serve. If making an omelette for one, 4 egg whites are recommended, using an 8"-10" skillet. Top if desired, see *Toppings for Egg Dishes*.

Alternatives: When using previously prepared chili, spaghetti sauce or manicotti filling, place desired amount in bowl and heat in microwave or in a small sauce pan. Place heated mixture on eggs as described above.

Philly-style Steak Omelette

This is a favorite in our household. It is a great recipe for leftover steak.

Sliced beef
Sliced onion
Sliced bell pepper

Egg whites
Grated nonfat cheese

If using leftover steak slices: Sauté onions and bell peppers over medium-high heat, until tender. Add steak slices and continue to cook until meat is warmed. Remove from pan and set aside.

If using raw beef: Slice meat thinly. Sauté meat, onions and bell peppers together over medium-high heat until vegetables are tender and steak is done to your liking. In either case, do not over cook steak, it will be too tough to chew. Remove from pan and set aside.

Prepare omelette shell as described in *Omelette* recipe. Put steak mixture over half of omelette, sprinkle with cheese. Fold other half of shell over filling, allow cheese to melt, serve.

Scrambled Eggs - Fancy

6 Egg whites

1 Cup any assortment of vegetables and/or meat (ham, ground turkey breast)

This is similar to the omlette recipe. The only difference is that you don't make an egg shell for the filling, just add the egg whites to the cooked filling and cook it all together until eggs are completely cooked through. The Denver omelette recipe will be used as an example for this *Scramble Egg - Fancy* recipe, other fillings can be used.

1/4 Cup chopped onions
1/4 Cup chopped bell peppers

1/2 Cup diced, lean ham
6 Egg whites
Dash of **Tabasco sauce** (optional)

Blend egg whites and Tabasco sauce in small bowl, set aside. Coat skillet with non-stick cooking spray, preheat over medium-high heat. Add onions, bell peppers and ham, cook for 8-10 minutes until vegetables are tender and ham is browned. Pour in egg whites and cook for approximately 7-10 minutes or until eggs are cooked all the way through. Stir mixture frequently to prevent sticking and burning. There you go! Scramble egg whites with your favorite flavors. Top if desired, see *Toppings for Egg Dishes*.

Egg Hash

If you've mastered the *Scrambled Eggs-Fancy* you are ready to take on this recipe.

Serves 2-3

6 Egg whites
1 Cup diced cooked potato
1/2 Cup diced onion

1/4 lb. Lean ground turkey breast
1/4 Cup barbecue sauce
Pepper/herbs to taste (optional)

Blend egg whites in small bowl, set aside. If you don't have any leftover potatoes, quickly cook up a potato or two in the microwave and dice. Coat skillet with non-stick cooking spray and preheat over medium-high heat. Crumble ground turkey in skillet, cook until half done, 4-6 minutes. Add diced potato and onion, continue to cook over medium-high heat until turkey is cooked and onions are tender. Stir in barbecue sauce, cook 2-3 more minutes. Pour in egg whites and cook until egg whites are fully cooked, turning frequently to prevent sticking and burning. Serve with toast, biscuits or muffins.

Alternatives: Add chopped celery or bell peppers.

Breakfast Burritos

Make filling the same as directed in *Scrambled Eggs - Fancy*. Use 2-3 egg whites per person.

Egg Whites
Your choice of diced fillings

Whole wheat tortillas

Lay tortillas on foil sprayed with non-stick cooking spray, cover tortillas completely with foil. Place in 250 degree oven and let warm for about 20 minutes (3-5 tortillas). The more tortillas you are heating the longer they will take to warm.

Cook fillings as instructed in *Scrambled Egg - Fancy*; Pre-cook diced fillings until tender. Pour in egg whites and cook until eggs are well-done. Place a couple of spoonfuls of mixture onto warm tortilla. If desired, sprinkle with cheese. Roll tortilla and place seam side down on plate. Top with your favorite topping, see *Toppings for Egg Dishes*. You can eat these with your hands by putting desired toppings in burrito instead of on top.

Breakfast Tostada

This is a very attractive dish and easy to prepare for a large brunch gathering.

Corn or whole wheat tortillas
1/4-1/2 Cup nonfat grated cheese
   per tortilla
Green onions, chopped
Turkey bacon, chopped (optional)

Egg whites (2-3 per tortilla
   depending on size of tortilla)
Bell peppers, sliced long and thin
Tomatoes, sliced long and thin

Toppings:
Nonfat sour cream and salsa

Preheat oven to 450 degrees. Coat cookie sheet with non-stick cooking spray. Quickly dip tortillas in water just until all of tortilla has been dampened, place flat on cookie sheet being careful not to overlap. Cook corn tortillas for 3-4 minutes, flour tortillas for 4-5 minutes, until light brown. Remove from oven and arrange cheese, onions and turkey bacon evenly in circle along outside edges of tortilla. Place two or more egg whites in center of cheese circle. Make sure tortilla edges are completely covered with the cheese and egg to prevent further browning. Bake until eggs are cooked thoroughly, 5-7 minutes for two eggs. Garnish with bell peppers, onions and toppings of your choice. If you desire the onions and bell peppers more tender, place on top of egg whites before baking.

Easy Quiche

This recipe is so easy and tasty even men will eat this quiche! Because there is no crust, this dish is very lean. You could always substitute the ham and onions with equaling amounts of broccoli, spinach, Canadian bacon, turkey bacon, bell peppers, mushrooms, zucchini, the list goes on. Put in whatever you like.

1 Cup egg whites
   (approx. 8 large eggs)
1 Cup water
3 Tbls. corn meal
1/2 Cup lowfat biscuit mix
1/2 Cup instant nonfat powdered
   dry milk

1/2 Cup nonfat sour cream
3/4 Cup diced onion
1 Cup shredded nonfat cheese
1 Cup diced, lean ham
Sour cream (optional)

Preheat oven to 350 degrees. Spray deep 9" pie plate with non-stick cooking spray.

Place first 6 ingredients into food processor or blender and blend for about 45 seconds. Batter should be very smooth. In medium size bowl combine batter mixture with ham, cheese and onions. Stir with spoon until well blended. Pour into pie plate. Bake for 40 - 50 minutes or until middle is set (middle doesn't jiggle). Let stand and cool for 10 minutes before serving. Top with nonfat sour cream. Most any carbohydrate side dish will compliment this dish; potatoes, pancakes, toast, muffins, biscuits or bowl of fruit.

Breakfast Potatoes

Fried Mashed Potatoes

These would make a great side dish for dinner as well.

Left over mashed potatoes.

Coat pan with non-stick cooking spray. Spoon desired amount of potatoes into pan. Break up any large chunks. Cook potatoes over medium-high heat turning frequently to prevent burning. Cook until thoroughly warmed and outer layers are golden brown.

Variations: Before putting potatoes in pan, dice any one of the following ingredients; onions, celery, garlic, bell peppers and cook until tender. Re-coat pan with non-stick cooking spray, add potatoes and proceed with cooking as instructed above.

Hash Browns

There is quite a variety of fat free, low sodium frozen potato products on the market. Try different brands to find the potatoes you like best. To make cooking time quick, cook frozen potatoes in microwave, on high, for 4 minutes per plateful. Coat large skillet or griddle with non-stick cooking spray, heat over medium-high heat. Cook potatoes until golden brown on the outside and steaming hot on the inside.

Fried Diced Potatoes

Left over baked potatoes, or raw potatoes.

If potatoes are raw, cooked desired amount of potatoes in microwave. Let cool for 10 minutes.

Dice or slice cooked potatoes into 1/4"-1/2" size. Coat pan with non-stick spray and place potatoes in pan. Cook over medium-high heat tossing potatoes until brown on all sides. Remove and serve when done to your liking.

Variations: Dice any of the following ingredients; onions, celery, garlic, bell peppers and cook right along with potatoes until potatoes are done and vegetables are tender. Turning frequently to prevent burning.

Muffins

Cinnamon Apple

Banana Cornmeal

Pumpkin Bran

Banana Blueberry

Blueberry

All of the following muffins have been baked in a large muffin pan. If smaller muffins are desired decrease oven temperature to 350 degrees and reduce cooking time by five to ten minutes. These muffin recipes may be cut in half or doubled.

Cinnamon Apple Muffins

1 1/2 Cups whole wheat flour
1/2 Cup **bran, unflaked**
1/3 Cup sugar or equivalent amount of artificial sweetener*
1 tsp. Cinnamon
1 Tbls. baking powder
1 Cup nonfat milk, or equal amount of evaporated skimmed milk
1/2 Cup unsweetened applesauce
2 Egg whites, slightly beaten
1 Cup baking apple, peeled and chopped

* See equivalents on sweetener product you choose to use.

Preheat oven to 400 degrees. Coat large muffin pan with non-stick cooking spray.

In a large mixing bowl blend together dry ingredients; set aside. In a separate bowl combine remaining ingredients, blend well with spoon or whisk. Pour wet mixture into dry ingredients and stir just until dry ingredients are moistened.

Fill muffin cups 3/4 full and bake for 25-30 minutes, makes 5 large muffins. To check doneness insert wooden toothpick into center of muffin, if toothpick comes out clean muffins are done. If muffin tops are becoming too brown, before centers are thoroughly cooked, cover with foil and return to oven.

When muffins are done baking, remove pan from oven and let cool for 10 minutes. Remove muffins from pan and set on cooling rack until completely cooled. Store in an airtight container or wrap individually. The muffins may be frozen.

Banana Cornmeal Muffins

2 Cups whole wheat flour
1 1/2 Cups cornmeal
1/3 Cup of sugar or equivalent amount of amount of artificial sweetener *
2 Tbls. baking powder
1/4 tsp. Nutmeg

1 3/4 Cups mashed very ripe bananas, (approximately 3)
1 Cup nonfat milk, or equal amount of evaporated skimmed milk
4 Egg whites, slightly beaten
1 Cup unsweetened applesauce

* See equivalents on sweetener product you choose to use.

Preheat oven to 400 degrees. Coat large muffin pan with non-stick cooking spray.

In a large mixing bowl blend together dry ingredients; set aside. In a separate bowl combine remaining ingredients, blend well with spoon or whisk. Pour wet mixture into dry ingredients and stir just until dry ingredients are moistened.

Fill muffin cups 3/4 full and bake for 25-30 minutes, makes 9 large muffins. To check doneness insert wooden toothpick into center of muffin, if toothpick comes out clean, muffins are done. If muffin tops are becoming too brown, before centers are thoroughly cooked, cover with foil and return to oven.

When muffins are done baking, remove pan from oven and let cool for 10 minutes. Remove muffins from pan and set on cooling rack until completely cooled. Store in an airtight container or wrap individually. The muffins may be frozen.

Pumpkin Bran Muffins

2 Cups wheat bran cereal, not flaked
1 Cup undiluted, evaporated skimmed milk
3 Cups whole wheat flour
1/2 Cup of sugar or equivalent amount of artifical sweetener *
2 Tbls. baking powder
2 tsp. Cinnamon
1 tsp. Nutmeg
1/4 tsp. **Ground cloves** or allspice
2 Cups pumpkin
1 1/2 Cups unsweetened applesauce
1/2 Cup apple juice concentrate
4 Egg whites, slightly beaten
1 Cup raisins (optional)

* See equivalents on sweetener product you choose to use.

Preheat oven to 400 degrees. Coat large muffin pan with non-stick cooking spray.

In medium sized mixing bowl combine wheat bran cereal and evaporated skimmed milk, stir until cereal is moistened; set aside.

In a large mixing bowl blend together next six dry ingredients; set aside. In a separate bowl combine remaining ingredients, blend well with spoon or whisk. our wet mixture into cereal mixture and stir until well blended. Pour this mixture into dry ingredients and stir just until dry ingredients are moistened.

Fill muffin cups 3/4 full and bake for 30-35 minutes, makes 11 large muffins. To check doneness insert wooden toothpick into center of muffin, if toothpick comes out clean, muffins are done. If muffin tops are becoming too brown, before centers are thoroughly cooked, cover with foil and return to oven.

When muffins are done baking, remove pan from oven and let cool for 10 minutes. Remove muffins from pan and set on cooling rack until completely cooled. Store in an airtight container or wrap individually. The muffins may be frozen.

Banana Blueberry Muffins

2 1/2 Cups whole wheat flour
1/3 Cup of sugar or equivalent
   amount of artificial sweetener *
2 Tbls. Baking powder
1/4 tsp. Nutmeg
3/4 Cup nonfat milk or equal amount
   of evaporated skimmed milk

3/4 Cup **nonfat buttermilk**
1/2 Cup unsweetened applesauce
1 Very ripe banana, mashed
4 Egg whites, slightly beaten
1 tsp. **Almond extract**
1 tsp. **Lemon Juice**
2 Cups **blueberries**, fresh or frozen

* See equivalents on sweetener product you choose to use.

Preheat oven to 400 degrees. Coat large muffin pan with non-stick cooking spray.

In a large mixing bowl blend together first four dry ingredients; set aside. In a separate bowl combine remaining ingredients, except blueberries, blend well with spoon or whisk. Pour wet mixture into dry mixture and stir until well blended. Gently fold in blueberries, do not overmix to keep blueberries plump.

Fill muffin cups 3/4 full and bake for 30-35 minutes, makes 8 large muffins. To check doneness insert wooden toothpick into center of muffin, if toothpick comes out clean, muffins are done. If muffin tops are becoming too brown, before centers are thoroughly cooked, cover with foil and return to oven.

When muffins are done baking, remove pan from oven and let cool for 10 minutes. Remove muffins from pan and set on cooling rack until completely cooled. Store in an airtight container or wrap individually. The muffins may be frozen.

Blueberry Muffins

1 1/2 Cups **blueberries**, fresh or frozen
2 Tbls. sugar or equivalent
    amount of artificial sweetener *

2 2/3 Cup whole wheat flour
1/4 Cup sugar or equivalent
    amount of artificial sweetener *
1 Tbls. plus, 1/2 tsp. Baking powder

1 Cup nonfat milk or equal amount
    of evaporated skimmed milk
4 Egg whites, slightly beaten
3/4 Cup unsweetened applesauce

* See equivalents on sweetener product you choose to use.

Preheat oven to 375 degrees. Coat large muffin pan with non-stick cooking spray.

In small mixing bowl gently stir sweetener and berries together, set aside.

In a large mixing bowl blend together next three 0dry ingredients; set aside. In a separate bowl combine remaining ingredients, blend well with spoon or whisk. Pour wet mixture into dry ingredients and stir just until dry ingredients are moistened. Gently fold in blueberries, do not overmix to keep blueberries plump.

Fill muffin cups 3/4 full and bake for 25-30 minutes, makes 6 large muffins. To check doneness insert wooden toothpick into center of muffin, if toothpick comes out clean, muffins are done. If muffin tops are becoming too brown, before centers are thoroughly cooked, cover with foil and return to oven.

When muffins are done baking, remove pan from oven and let cool for 10 minutes. Remove muffins from pan and set on cooling rack until completely cooled. Store in an airtight container or wrap individually. The muffins may be frozen.

Lunch

Sandwiches:
Egg Salad
Tuna Salad
Chicken or Turkey Salad
Egg and Tuna Salad
Barbecue Beef
Barbecue Pork
Philly-style Steak

Soups:
Chicken or Turkey
Vegetable Beef
Clam Chowder

Sandwiches

Egg Salad Sandwich
Tuna Salad Sandwich
Chicken or Turkey Salad Sandwich
Egg/Tuna Salad Sandwich

All of these sandwiches are made in the same manner, the only difference is the main ingredient which could be egg whites, tuna, chicken, turkey, or any combination.

Main ingredient: 1- 12 oz. Can water-packed, chunk light tuna, drained, **or**
1 - 12 oz. Can water-packed, chunk light chicken meat, drained, **or**
6 - 8 Hard-boiled egg whites, grated or chopped, **or**
2 Cups left over chicken or turkey breast, chunked, **or**
1 - 6 oz. Can water-packed, chunk light tuna, drained, plus 4 grated egg whites

Whole wheat bread slices
1/4-1/2 Cup nonfat mayonnaise
1 Tbls. Dijon mustard
1/4 Cup chopped celery
1/4 Cup chopped sweet or dill pickles, or 2 Tbls. prepared relish
1/4 Cup chopped green onion
Tomato slices and lettuce (optional)

Makes 2-3 sandwiches

Place main ingredient in medium-sized bowl. Break up large chunks with fork. Add onion, celery, and pickles, stir with fork. Add mayonnaise and mustard, stir until well blended. Add more mayonnaise or mustard if desired. Spread onto one slice of bread as thin or thick as you like, add sliced tomato and piece of lettuce, sandwich with other slice of bread and there you have it. For open-faced sandwich, lay lettuce and tomato slices on bread, spoon sandwich filling on top, do not sandwich with second piece of bread. You may also toast the bread.

Barbecue Beef Sandwich
or
Barbecue Pork Sandwich

This one is so easy it's embarrassing.

Whole wheat bread slices, or whole wheat hamburger buns	Nonfat mayonnaise
	Mustard
Leftover eye of round roast, pork loin roast or boneless spare ribs	Onions, sliced
	Tomato slices
Barbecue sauce	Lettuce

Shred beef or pork into small, microwavable mixing bowl. If shredded pieces of meat are too long (2+ inches) cut into smaller bite-sized lengths. That way one bite won't wipe out the entire sandwich of most of its meat. Add enough barbecue sauce to moisten the meat without making it too soupy. Heat in microwave oven or in a sauce pan, just until warmed, it doesn't have to be hot.

While meat is heating, toast bread slices and coat with mustard or mayonnaise if desired. Add sliced onions, tomato and lettuce for a real treat. The sliced onions can also be combined with the meat and heated together. Spoon desired amount onto bread, serve with beans or fruit salad.

Philly-style Steak Sandwich

This is a great way to use up any left-over steak.

Leftover steak, thinly sliced (enough for number of sandwiches you plan to make)	Whole wheat rolls, buns or bread
	Nonfat cheese, grated or sliced
	Dijon mustard
Bell pepper thinly sliced	Nonfat mayonnaise
Medium onion, thinly sliced	

Spray skillet with non-stick cooking spray, heat over medium-high heat. Sauté bell pepper and onion slices until they become tender. Add steak and cook just until steak is warmed, you do not want to overcook the steak. Sprinkle with grated cheese or lay cheese slices on warmed meat and vegetables, allow cheese to melt. Remove from heat and set aside. Toast bread under broiler until golden brown, spread on mustard and mayonnaise, add steak mixture and enjoy. If using sliced bread, toast bread in toaster.

Soups

Chicken or Turkey Soup

Soup is very easy to make and the ingredients are versatile. Any combination of the following ingredients can be used or feel free to add to the ingredients.

2 - 49 1/2 oz. Cans reduced sodium chicken broth
3-4 Boneless, skinless chicken breast, cooked and chunked or shredded, **or**
2 - 12oz. cans water packed chunk light chicken undrained, **or**
1-2 Turkey breast, cooked, and chunked or shredded

1/4 Cup **barley**
1 Cup chopped onion
1 Cup thinly sliced carrots
1 Cup diced celery
1/2 Cup chopped broccoli
2 Cups diced potatoes or 3 Cups **no-yolk egg noodles**

In large soup pot or crock pot combine all ingredients except for onions and pasta. Cook over medium heat until potatoes become tender. Crock pot should be set on high. Simmer for 1-2 hours. Increase heat to medium, add onion and pasta and cook for an additional 10-15 minutes, or until pasta is tender. Serve. This soup can be frozen.

Vegetable Beef Soup

Use the beef leftover from an eye of round roast or boneless spare ribs.

2 - 49 1/2 oz. Cans beef broth
3-4 Cups beef, cooked, shredded or chunked
1 Cup corn, drained
1 Cup string beans, canned or fresh, drained

2 Cups diced red potatoes
1 - 15 oz. Can reduced sodium kidney beans, drained
1 - 14 1/2 oz. Can stewed tomatoes chopped

In large soup pot or crock pot combine all ingredients and cook over medium heat, bringing soup to a low boil. Crock pot heat should be set on high. Cook until potatoes become tender, serve. Soup can simmer for 1-2 hours if desired. This soup can be frozen.

Clam Chowder

2 - 6 1/2 oz. Cans **minced clams**, add another can if you like it real clammy
2 Cups potatoes, diced 1/2"-1" (red, white, russet or any combination)
3 Cups chopped onion
1 Cup chopped celery
1/4-1/2 Cup chopped celery leaves
4 Slices turkey bacon, finely chopped **or** 1/2 cup finely diced ham

1 - 8 oz. Jar **clam juice**
1 Cup water
1/2 tsp. **Dried thyme**
Ground pepper to taste
1 **Bay leaf**
4 sprigs **fresh parsley**
1/4 Cup all purpose flour or *Wondra*
2 Cups evaporated skimmed milk

Drain clams saving juice, set aside. Cook turkey bacon or ham until crisp, place on paper towel; set aside.

Coat large skillet with non-stick cooking spray, heat over medium-high heat. Cook potatoes, onion, celery and celery leaves together for 8-10 minutes. Turn to prevent burning and sticking. Stir in turkey bacon or ham, cook for an additional 2 minutes. Transfer to large soup pot. Add clam juice (jar and reserve from cans), water and next four ingredients. Cook over medium heat bringing to a slow boil, reduce heat to simmer, cover and cook for 15-20 minutes or until potatoes are tender. Remove parsley and bay leaf.

With flour in small bowl, gradually add milk stirring constantly until flour is completely blended and mixture is smooth. Stir flour mixture into soup. Increase cooking temperature to medium, cook for an additional 10-15 minutes until soup thickens, stirring frequently. Add clams, reduce heat to simmer and cook another 5 minutes.

Dinner

Crock Pot Dinners:
Turkey Breast
Turkey Breast Tenderloin
Pork Loin Roast
Boneless Pork Chops
Boneless Pork Spareribs
Eye of Round Beef Roast
Boneless Beef Spareribs
Stewed Beef
With Gravy!

Family Favorites:
Chicken or Turkey Stroganoff
Kebabs for All, With Polynesian Sauce
Turkey Meatloaf or Meatballs

Chili:
Turkey Chili
Chili Casserole

Mexican Dishes:
Quesadilla
Tostada
Soft Tacos
Burritos
Nachos

Italian and Pasta Dishes:
Lasagna
Pizza
Spaghetti Meat Sauce
Quick and Easy Spaghetti Meat Sauce
Manicotti

Vegetable Dishes:
Stuffed Cabbage Rolls
Stuffed Bell Peppers

Crock Pot Dinners

**Turkey Breast, or
Turkey Breast Tenderloins, or
Pork Loin Roast, or
Boneless Pork Chops, or
Boneless Pork Spareribs
<u>With gravy!</u>**

Because of the ability to make gravy from this dinner it is a winner when served with mashed potatoes and vegetables. The amount of meat you use depends on how many you plan to serve, how many leftovers you want and the size of your crock pot.

1-3 lbs. Turkey or Pork; whole turkey breast **or** turkey breast tenderloins **or**, pork loin roast **or**, large boneess pork chops **or,** lean pork spareribs

2 - 14 1/2 oz. Cans reduced sodium chicken broth

1 Small onion, cut into fours

1 Bell pepper, small, deseeded, cut into fours

1-3 whole garlic cloves, peeled, cut in half

Celery stalk, with leaves, cut into 3" peices

Wondra, gray thickener (recipe to follow)

Place onion, bell peppers, garlic and celery into crock pot. Trim off any excess fat from pork or remove skin on turkey, add to crock pot. Cover meat and vegetables with broth. If broth does not cover add water until food is completely covered. Cook on high for 4-8 hours. Turn to low heat until you are ready to serve. Just before serving, prepare gravy.

Gravy: Using a baster or deep spoon, carefully remove clear liquid, place in small sauce pan. Cook over medium-high heat to a medium boil. Allow *Wondra* to pour out slowly through small holes in container while simultaneously stirring quickly until desired thickness is acquired. Gravy tends to thicken a little bit more as it cooks. Cover and simmer until ready to serve.

Eye of Round Beef Roast, or Boneless Beef Spare Ribs or Stewed Beef <u>*With Gravy!*</u>

The amount of meat you use depends on how many you plan to serve, how many leftovers you want and the size of your crock pot.

- 1-3 lbs. Eye of Round roast or lean boneless beef spareribs or stew meat
- 2 - 14 1/2 oz. Cans beef broth
- 1-3 Whole garlic cloves, peeled, cut in half

- 3-5 Small red potatoes, cut in half
- 3-4 Carrots, peeled, cut in thirds

- 1 Onion, small, cut into fours
- 1 Bell pepper, small, de-seeded, cut into fours
- Celery stalk with leaves, cut into 3" pieces
- *Wondra*, gravy thickener (recipe to follow)

Place onion, bell peppers, garlic and celery into crock pot. Trim off any excess fat on meat, add to crock pot.* Cover meat and vegetables with broth. If broth does not cover add water until food is completely covered. Cook on high for 4-8 hours. Add small potatoes and carrots 40-45 minutes before serving. Ready to serve when potatoes are tender. Turn heat to low until you are ready to serve. Just before serving, prepare gravy.

* Optional step: In large skillet coated with non-stick cooking spray, brown meat on all sides over medium-high heat. Remove from heat and place in crock pot with vegetables.

Gravy: Using a baster or deep spoon, carefully remove clear liquid, place in small sauce pan. Cook over medium-high heat to a medium boil. Allow *Wondra* to pour out slowly through small holes in container while simultaneously stirring quickly until desired thickness is acquired. Gravy tends to thicken a little bit more as it cooks. Cover and simmer until ready to serve.

Family Favorites

Chicken or Turkey Stroganoff

4 Chicken breast halves, boneless, skinless **or**, two medium-sized turkey breast tenderloins
2 Cups sliced onion and/or bell pepper
3 Cups sliced mushrooms (appx. 1/2 lb.)
2/3 Cup low sodium chicken broth
2 Tbls. *Wondra*, for thickening
2 tsp. Paprika
3 Minced garlic cloves, or 1 tsp. garlic powder (optional)
1 Cup chopped stewed tomatoes
1/2 Cup nonfat sour cream

Slice chicken or turkey breast into 1/4" strips. Spray large skillet with non-stick cooking spray, preheat over medium-high heat. Cook meat 5-8 minutes. Add onions, bell peppers and mushrooms, cook until vegetables are tender and meat is completely cooked. Reduce heat to warm, stir in garlic and paprika. In small cup or bowl, blend broth and *Wondra* until smooth, stir into meat and vegetable mixture. Add in tomatoes and sour cream, stir until well blended. Cook at low boil for 10-15 minutes, stir occasionally. Serve over diced potatoes, no-yolk egg noodles, mashed potatoes or bed of brown rice.

Time saving idea: If you like to buy your mushrooms whole, rinse clean then slice mushrooms with egg slicer.

Alternative: To make beef stroganoff use two pounds lean top sirloin or London Broil, and use 2/3 cup beef broth instead of chicken broth. Slice thinly and cook as directed above.

Kebabs for All

Have a kebab barbecue party! You can supply the barbecue, skewers and ingredients. Have the guest supply salads and side dishes, or have guests supply one or more of the kebab ingredients. Everyone can create their own kebabs using the ingredients they like most.

Supplies: Wooden or wire skewers (wire skewers can be hot to the touch, be careful). Be sure to soak wooden skewers in water for 10-15 minutes before using, this will help prevent burning of the skewers.

        Barbecue or oven

Ingredients (to be cut into 1" - 1 1/2" bite-sized pieces):

Meats:	Chicken breast Turkey breast **Shrimp/prawns**	Lean beef (sirloin) Fish (shark, swordfish, halibut, tuna) Turkey bacon to wrap around vegetables
Vegetables:	Bell peppers Mushrooms Potatoes Carrots **Cauliflower**	Onions **Cherry tomatoes** **Corn on the cob,** sliced Broccoli Zucchini
Fruits:	Pineapple	Apples
Sauces:	**Teriyaki** **Lemon and herb**	Barbecue **Polynesian** (recipe to follow)

You may need to pre-cook the carrots and potatoes just a bit so they come out tender after barbecuing or baking. Put pieces on plate, cover with paper towel, cook in microwave, on high for 5-8 minutes, just until tender. They will continue to cook on grill or in the oven.

Fill skewers with your choice of meats, vegetables and/or fruit. Place prepared skewers on grill and barbecue on medium heat, turning every 8-10 minutes until meat is thoroughly cooked. If you are using an oven, cook kebabs under a broiler 5-8 minutes on each side. Rack may have to be lowered one tier so food does not burn.

Alternatives: Serve kebabs over bed of brown/wild rice or cous cous (pasta).

Polynesian Sauce

This sauce is especially good on pork and poultry.

1 Cup undiluted apple juice concentrate	1 - 8 oz. Can **crushed pineapple,** undrained
4 Tbls. cornstarch	1/4 Cup minced onion
1/4 Cup **low sodium soy sauce**	1 Tbls. **Worcestershire**
1/2 Cup water	1 Tbls. **freshly grated ginger** or 1 tsp. **dry ginger**
1/3 Cup **apple cider vinegar**	
1 Tbls. **grated orange rind** (or finely chop)	1/4 Cup of sugar or equivalent amount of artificial sweetener *

* See equivalents on sweetener product you choose to use.

Put cornstarch in small bowl or cup. Gradually add apple juice, stirring frequently until well blended and smooth. Pour into medium-sized sauce pan. Add remaining ingredients and stir. (Except artificial sweetener; okay to add sugar here). Cook over medium heat until sauce begins to thicken, stir frequently. Cook until desired thickness, 5-7 minutes. Let cool for 30 minutes. If using artificial sweetener, stir in after sauce has cooled 30 minutes. Brush sauce onto kebabs as they are cooking or use as a dip.

Turkey Meatloaf or Meatballs

1 1/2 - 2 lbs. Lean ground turkey breast
1/2 Cup finely chopped onion
1/2 Cup finely chopped water chestnuts
1 - 8 oz. Can stewed tomatoes, drained and chopped
1/3 Cup barbecue sauce
1/2 Cup Oatmeal, or seasoned bread crumbs or 1/2 cup combination of the two
4 Egg whites
1/2 tsp. Italian herb blend

Meatloaf:
Place all ingredients in large bowl. With two-pronged fork or your hands, blend ingredients together. Try not to over blend as this will make the meatloaf a little mushy. In bowl, form meat mixture into ball. Place ball in shallow baking pan that has been coated with non-stick cooking spray, form into an oblong-shaped loaf. (A cookie sheet or holeless pizza pan would work too.) Bake at 375 degrees for 1 hour to 1 hour and fifteen minutes. These can also be divided into two bread pans. Coat with non-stick cooking spray and bake for 40-50 minutes. To test for doneness, after one hour of baking, push on top of meatloaf with utensil or finger. If meat feels very firm the meatloaf should be cooked thoroughly. If meat feel mushy or springs back, continue baking and recheck every ten minutes.

Meatballs:
To make meatballs, simply shape mixture into 2" balls. Cook in large skillet coated with non-stick cooking spray over medium-heat. Turn meatballs to brown on all sides. Cook for approximately 20 minutes, or until meat is thoroughly cooked.

Time saver tip: If only serving one or two, cook half of the mixture as a meatloaf and form meatballs from the other half and freeze them for later use. Or, freeze the other half to make another meatloaf at a later time.

Chili

Turkey Chili

You can make a lot of chili in a short amount of time. Freeze in small containers for a handy lunch meal. This recipe can easily be cut in half.

- 1 1/2 to 2 lbs. Lean ground turkey breast
- 2 Bell peppers, any combination of green, red or yellow, diced into 1/2" pieces
- 2 Medium onion, yellow or white, diced into 1/2 pieces
- 2 - 15 oz. Cans black beans, drained
- 2 - 15 oz. Cans kidney beans, low sodium, drained
- 1-2 Cans water
- 2 - 15 oz. Cans chili seasoned pinto beans
- 2 - 14 1/2 oz. Cans chili seasoned chunky tomato sauce, or Mexican seasoned stewed tomatoes, chopped
- 1 - 12 oz. Can tomato paste
- 2 Packages specialty * chili seasoning mixes (or see below for seasonings to use from a well stocked spice cabinet)

* *2 Alarm Chili Kit* or *Carroll Shelby Chili Mix* (Sodium content is high due to separate salt packet, omit the salt). These two brand names should be available at your local grocery store. Also, use only 1 1/2 of the large chili powder seasoning packets from these mixes. Add the remaining seasonings to your spice cabinet.

You will need one large skillet and one large pot (6+ quarts). Coat both with non-stick cooking spray. In skillet, crumble turkey burger into small chunks and cook over medium-high heat until cooked thoroughly. Break up any large pieces with spoon or spatula while cooking. When done pour meat into pot, set aside. In same skillet, spray another coat of non-stick cooking spray, add chopped bell peppers and onion and cook just until tender, but not too limp. These vegetables will continue to cook while the chili is simmering to perfection. Pour into pot with turkey. The hard part is over.

Open all cans of beans and empty beans into pot with meat. Open remaining cans of tomato sauce and paste, add to pot. I often put water in the tomato cans as a way to rinse them out reserving the water for the chili. Add one can of water and stir with large spoon. Add all chili seasonings and spices, except for salt, red pepper and masa flour. Discard salt and decide whether or not you want to add the red pepper. If you like really hot and spicy chili add the whole packet, add just a little bit if you like your chili on the medium side, and don't add it at all if you prefer mild chili. Stir until well blended. Add more water only if chili seems too thick (as it simmers it becomes thinner, you don't want it too soupy to begin with). Simmer chili, uncovered, on stove top for 1-2 hours or in the oven at 275 degrees for same amount of time stirring, occasionally. Just before serving or putting in containers to freeze, prepare masa flour as directed (see below) and stir into the chili. Serve with cornbread, or banana cornmeal muffins (see recipe).

Home-made chili seasonings for this recipe:

1/2 Cup chili powder	1 Tbls. cumin
1 Tbls. **minced garlic**	2 tsp. **Oregano**, crushed leaves
1 Tbls. paprika	**Red pepper or cayenne pepper** to taste
	2 Tbls. **Masa corn flour**

Masa corn flour instructions. Put flour into small cup. Gradually pour in 1/4-1/2 cup of water stirring constantly. Stir until all flour is moistened and mixture is thick but pourable. Add to chili and stir until well blended, ready to serve.

Chili Casserole

I can't decide which I like better, this easy chili casserole or turkey chili, you decide. I make this recipe in large quantities to ensure many lunches, a couple of dinners and an omelette or two. You may freeze the leftovers or cut the recipe in half.

2 lbs. Lean ground turkey breast
2 Cups diced onion
2 Cups diced bell peppers
2 Cups whole kernel corn, drained
1 Tbls. ground cumin
1 tsp. Garlic powder
1 Tbls. plus 1 tsp. chili powder
2 - 16 oz. Cans chili seasoned beans
2 - 14 1/2 oz. Cans Mexican seasoned stewed tomatoes, undrained and chopped
1 - 12 oz. Can tomato paste
1 - 4 oz. plus 1 - 7 oz. Can chopped or diced green chilies
1 Cup water (more if you like it soupy, less if you like it thicker)
Shredded nonfat cheese

Preheat oven to 350 degrees. Coat large casserole dish or small roasting pan with non-stick cooking spray.

In large skillet crumble ground turkey, cook over medium heat until thoroughly done. Place cooked turkey in large mixing bowl. Next, cook onion and bell peppers until vegetables are tender but not too limp, add to meat mixture. Add rest of ingredients except for water, stir until well blended. Gradually add water to reach desired consistency, remembering that mixture will become more soupy as it cooks. Pour into prepared dish, cover and bake for 30-40 minutes. Serve hot, sprinkled with nonfat cheese. Great served with cornbread or banana cornmeal muffins (see recipe). Leftovers make a great lunch. This chili is also good served over diced baked potatoes, mashed potatoes, rice or as an omelette filling.

Mexican Dishes

Quesadilla

Main ingredients:
    Corn or whole wheat flour tortillas (fat free if possible)
    Shredded nonfat cheese
    Non-stick cooking spray

Additions:
    Diced onion   Salsa
    Diced bell pepper   Shredded meat or poultry
    Nonfat refried beans   Nonfat sour cream

Coat large skillet with non-stick cooking spray, heat over medium heat. Lightly coat one side of tortilla with vegetable spray, place sprayed side down in pan. Sprinkle cheese to cover tortilla. Add 1-2 tablespoons of any additional ingredients. Spray another tortilla with non-stick cooking spray, place sprayed side up over first tortilla and fillings. Cook until cheese is melted and tortilla is golden brown on both sides. Remove from heat and let cool for 2-3 minutes. Cut in half, quarters or six equal triangles.

Tostada

4-6 Corn or flour tortillas
1 - 15 oz. Can nonfat refried beans
1 lb. Lean ground turkey breast, or
3-4 Boneless, skinless chicken breast cooked, cooled, shredded or chunked
1 Small pkt. taco seasoning (optional)
1 Cup chopped green onions

1 - 4 oz. Can diced green chilies
1 Cup shredded nonfat cheese
1 Cup chopped tomatoes
2 Cups shredded cabbage or lettuce
Nonfat sour cream
Salsa

Preheat oven to 250 degrees.

For soft tortillas, quickly run tortillas under water. Stack tortillas and wrap together in foil sprayed with non-stick cooking spray. Place in oven for about 20 minutes. For crisp tortillas, quickly run tortillas under water, place on cookie sheet sprayed with non-stick cooking spray, be careful not to overlap. Bake for 10-15 minutes, until crisp and golden brown. Remove from oven, set aside.

Heat beans in small sauce pan over medium heat until warmed, reduce heat to low, or heat beans in a microwave oven. Spray large skillet with non-stick cooking spray, heat over medium-high heat. Cook meat until thoroughly done. Season meat with taco seasoning by sprinkling on meat and stirring in, or by following instructions on packet. Reduce heat to keep warm.

Place warmed tortilla on plate. Evenly divide ingredients and layer starting with beans, meat, green chilies, cheese, green onions, cabbage and tomatoes. Garnish with sour cream and salsa.

Soft Tacos

6-8 Whole wheat tortillas, fat free if possible
1 lb. Lean ground turkey breast
1 Small pkt. Taco seasonings
1 Cup chopped green onions

1 Cup shredded nonfat cheese
1 Cup chopped tomatoes
2 Cups shredded cabbage or lettuce
Salsa
Nonfat sour cream

Preheat oven to 250 degrees.

Run tortillas quickly under water, stack, then wrap together in foil coated with non-stick cooking spray, and place in oven for about 20 minutes. Coat large skillet with non-stick cooking spray, heat over medium heat. Crumble and cook turkey until thoroughly done. Add taco seasoning to meat; follow directions on packet or just sprinkle over meat to add flavor. Reduce heat to low.

Remove tortillas from oven. Fold tortilla in half cupping in hand using a hot pad or place in tortilla holder. Layer starting with meat, green onions, cheese, tomatoes and cabbage or lettuce. Add a couple teaspoons of salsa and sour cream if desired.

Alternatives: If you have leftover beef, pork, chicken or turkey, shred meat and use in tacos. Season as directed above. Serve tacos with nonfat refried beans or put a layer of refried beans in taco, just before the meat.

Burritos

These can be made ahead of time and kept in the refrigerator until ready to bake and serve.

6-8 Whole wheat tortillas
4-6 Boneless, skinless chicken breast **or**, 2-3 small turkey breast tenderloins, **or** 1- 1 1/2 lbs. ground turkey breast
1 Small pkt. burrito seasonings
1 - 14 1/2 oz. Can Mexican seasoned stewed tomatoes, drained and chopped

1 Medium onion, thinly sliced
1 Bell pepper, thinly sliced
2 Cups **Spanish** or brown **rice** (optional)
2 Cups shredded cabbage or lettuce
Salsa
Nonfat sour cream

Preheat oven to 350 degrees. Heat refried beans in sauce pan or microwave, keep warm.

If you choose turkey tenderloins or chicken breast, slice into thin 1/4" strips. Coat large skillet with non-stick cooking spray, heat, over medium-high heat. Cook meat until half done. Add bell pepper and onion, continue to cook until meat is well done and vegetables are tender. Add burrito seasoning packet, following directions on packet, cook for 5-8 more minutes. Stir in chopped stewed tomatoes, remove from heat.

If you choose ground turkey breast, crumble and cook meat until half done. Add bell pepper and onion, continue to cook until meat is well done and vegetables are tender. Add burrito seasoning packet, following directions on packet, cook for 5-8 more minutes. Stir in chopped stewed tomatoes, remove from heat.

Set out one piece of foil for each tortilla, approximately 10"-12" in length. Lightly coat one side of foil with non-stick cooking spray; place tortilla in center of foil. Evenly divide and spread refried beans on each tortilla. Next, evenly divide meat mixture and place in center of tortillas. Do the same with the rice. Sprinkle on cheese. Roll tortilla into burrito, wrap foil completely around burrito. Place on cookie sheet and bake for 25-30 minutes. Remove from foil and garnish with salsa, cabbage or lettuce and nonfat sour cream. Burritos can also be heated in the microwave; wrap in moist paper towel and heat for 3 minutes. Garnish with cabbage or lettuce, salsa and sour cream.

Alternatives: If you have leftover beef, pork or poultry, shred meat and season as directed above.

Nachos

This dish can be made as a main course, an appetizer or a great party dish.

1 - 7-10 oz. Bag baked tortilla or corn chips, unsalted
1 - 15 oz. Can nonfat refried beans
1 lb. Lean ground turkey breast *
1 Small pkt. taco seasonings
1 - 7 oz. Can diced green chilies
1/2 Cup chopped green onions
2 Cups grated nonfat cheese (mozzarella is good for this recipe)
Fresh salsa
Nonfat sour cream

Preheat oven to 350 degrees.

To make four individual servings, use four large salad plates. To make one large serving use shallow baking dish or pizza pan. Lightly coat plates or pan with non-stick cooking spray.

Coat skillet with non-stick cooking spray, heat over medium-high heat. Crumble and cook ground turkey until thoroughly done. Season with seasoning packet as directed on package. Cook over medium heat until liquid is gone. Do not overcook meat, it will become too dry. Remove from heat.

Individual servings: Spread layer of chips on plates. Spoon small amounts of refried beans randomly on chips. Evenly disperse 1/4 cup seasoned meat and two tablespoons of green chilies and green onions over chips and beans. Cover with 1/4-1/2 cup grated cheese. You can stop here or layer again starting with chips. Warm in preheated oven for 15-20 or 20-25 minutes, one layer and two layers respectively. Check nachos periodically, if cheese or chips are browning too quickly, cover with foil. Serve with individual servings of salsa and sour cream or put in small bowls for everyone to serve themselves.

For one large serving: Make two layers beginning with chips. Spread half of the chips along bottom of pan. Spoon 1/2 can of refried beans in small amounts randomly on chips. Evenly disperse half of the meat, green chilies and green onions over chips and beans. Cover with one cup of grated cheese. Layer again starting with chips, ending with cheese. Warm in oven for 25-35 minutes. Check nachos periodically, if cheese or chips are browning too quickly, cover with foil. Serve with individual servings of salsa and sour cream or put in small bowls for everyone to serve themselves.

* If you have leftover beef roast, pork loin roast, turkey or chicken breast shred or chunk meat. Warm in skillet coated with non-stick spray over medium heat. Season meat as directed on seasoning packet, then proceed as directed.

Italian and Pasta Dishes

Lasagna

6-8 **Wide lasagna noodles,** cooked, drained, cooled *
2 lbs. Lean ground turkey breast
1 - 10 oz. Pkg. frozen spinach, thawed and squeezed to remove excess water

3 Cloves garlic, minced
2 - 27 1/2 oz. jars nonfat spaghetti sauce
1 Cup chopped onion
2 Cups nonfat cottage cheese
2 Cups shredded nonfat **mozzarella cheese**

* Available are lasagna noodles that don't need to be pre-cooked. They cook as lasagna is baking. Great time-saver.

Preheat oven to 350 degrees. Coat 9"x13" baking pan or dish with non-stick cooking spray.

Coat skillet with non-stick cooking spray, heat over medium-high heat. Crumble and cook ground turkey until half done. Add onions and garlic and continue to cook until turkey is thoroughly cooked and onions are tender. Stir in spaghetti sauce, bring to low boil. Reduce heat and let simmer for 10 minutes, stirring occasionally to prevent sticking.

Place 3-4 lasagna noodles evenly in bottom of pan. Layer starting with 1/2 meat sauce, 1/2 cottage cheese, 1/2 spinach and 1/2 mozzarella. Repeat layering. Cover and bake for 45-50 minutes, until thoroughly heated, edges will be bubbly. Uncover and bake for another 8-12 minutes, until cheese browns. Remove from oven and let cool for 15-20 minutes before serving.

Pizza

Prepared pizza crust (*Boboli*)
1/2 - 3/4 Cup pizza sauce, fat free or marinara

Following is a list of optional toppings:

Canadian bacon or ham	Pineapple
Ground turkey burger	Mushrooms
Chicken breast shredded	Zucchini slices
Bell peppers	Tomato slices
Onions	Nonfat grated cheese
Artichoke hearts (water packed)	

Preheat oven to 350 degrees.

Lightly coat bottom of pizza pan or large cookie sheet with non-stick cooking spray. Place crust on pan and coat with pizza sauce. Layer in the following order, pizza sauce or marinara, meat, vegetables, fruit, ending with cheese. Place on middle rack in oven and bake for 20-25 minutes. To ensure a crisp bottom crust, cook on bottom rack for first 12-15 minutes. Move to middle rack and continue to bake until cheese is golden brown, approximately another 10-12 minutes. Remove from oven, let cool for five minutes, slice and serve.

Spaghetti Meat Sauce

2 lbs. Lean ground turkey breast
1 Cup chopped onion
1 Cup sliced mushrooms
1 - 6 oz. can tomato paste

3 - 14 oz. Cans "Pasta" seasoned, chunky tomato sauce
1 Large packet spaghetti seasonings
1 Cup water

Coat large skillet with non-stick cooking spray, heat over medium heat. Crumble and cook ground turkey breaking up large chunks with spatula or spoon while cooking. When turkey is half done, add onions and mushrooms, continue to cook until vegetables are tender. Put mixture into large pot. Add tomato paste, chunky tomato sauce, seasoning packet and water. Stir and cook over medium heat until sauce begins to boil. Reduce heat and simmer for 30-45 minutes. Serve over your favorite pasta. You may freeze sauce in airtight containers.

Alternative: Pour sauce over cooked diced potatoes or use sauce as an omelette filling.

Quick and Easy Spaghetti Sauce

1 lb. Lean ground turkey breast
2 - 27 1/2 oz. jars nonfat spaghetti sauce
1 - 14 oz. can Italian seasoned chunky tomato sauce or stewed tomatoes, drained and chopped

Optional ingredients:
1 Cup chopped mushrooms
1 Cup chopped zucchini
1 Cup chopped onion

Coat large skillet with non-stick cooking spray, heat over medium heat. Crumble and cook ground turkey breaking up large chunks with spatula or spoon while cooking. When turkey is half done add optional ingredients, continue to cook until vegetables are tender. Put mixture into large pot. Add spaghetti sauce and chunky tomato sauce. Stir and cook over medium heat until sauce begins to boil. Reduce heat and simmer for 10 minutes. Serve over your favorite pasta. You may freeze sauce in airtight containers.

Manicotti

Referred to in this household as "Mazarattis".

Manicotti pasta, 12-14
  or **extra large pasta shells**
1 lb. Lean ground turkey breast
1 Medium onion, chopped
1 1/2 Cups kernel corn, drained
1 - 10 oz. Pkg. frozen, shopped spinach, thaw, squeeze out excess water

1 - 14 1/2 oz. Can chunky tomato sauce, Italian seasoned
1 Cup marinara or meatless spaghetti sauce
1 tsp. Italian herb blend
1 Cup nonfat grated cheese
Extra marinara sauce and cheese for topping

Preheat oven to 350 degrees.

Cook pasta according to directions on package, drain; set aside. You can prepare the whole package of pasta or just enough for a couple of servings. Any extra filling can be frozen and used at a later time or as a filling for your morning omelette.

Filling: Coat skillet with non-stick cooking spray. Crumble ground turkey and cook over medium-high heat until turkey is half done. Add onions, continue to cook until turkey is thoroughly cooked and onions are tender. In large mixing bowl add meat mixture and remaining ingredients, using only 1/2 cup of the cheese. Stir until well blended. If you desire a thicker tomato sauce mixture, add more marinara sauce.

Coat shallow baking pan or dish with non-stick cooking spray. Stuff pasta with filling being careful not to split shells. Use your hand or a pastry bag if you have one. Place stuffed shells in single layer in baking dish. Spread extra tomato sauce evenly over shells, sprinkle with remaining cheese, cover and bake for 30-35 minutes.

Vegetable Dishes

Stuffed Cabbage Rolls

1 lb. Lean ground turkey breast
4-6 Large cabbage leaves
1/2 Cup onion, chopped
1 Cup cooked brown rice
1 - 4 oz. Can diced green chilies
1 tsp. Italian herb seasoning

1 - 6 oz. can tomato paste
1 - 16 oz. can chopped tomatoes, undrained
1-2 Garlic cloves, minced
1 Egg white
1 Cup marinara sauce or tomato sauce

Preheat oven to 350 degrees. Coat medium sized baking dish with non-stick cooking spray.

Bring large pot of water to a boil. Carefully add one cabbage leaf at time, so as not to break them, and cook for 6-8 minutes or until wilted. Drain and set aside.

Coat large skillet with non-stick cooking spray, heat over medium-high heat. Crumble and cook ground turkey and onions until turkey is thoroughly cooked. Remove from heat and put in large mixing bowl. Add, rice, green chilies, tomato paste, chopped tomatoes, garlic, herbs and egg white. Stir until well blended. Depending on the size of your cabbage leaves place approximately 1/2 cup of filling onto cabbage leaf. Fold over the edges completely enclosing mixture. Place seam side down in baking dish. Pour marinara evenly over cabbage rolls. Cover and bake for 50-55 minutes.

Stuffed Bell Peppers

3-5 Whole bell peppers; green, yellow or red
1 lb. Lean ground turkey breast
1 Medium onion, chopped
1/2 Cup celery, chopped
1/2 Cup kernel corn, drained
1 Cup cooked barley or brown rice

1-2 15 oz. Cans chunky tomato sauce, Mexican seasoned
1 Tbls. chili powder
1/2 tsp. Cumin
1/2 tsp. **Oregano**, crushed leaves
1 Garlic clove minced, or 1/2 tsp. dry minced garlic, or 1/4 tsp. garlic powder
1/2 Cup Grated cheese (optional)

Preheat oven to 350 degrees.

Rinse bell peppers, cut off tops and clean out seeds and membrane. In large pot, large enough to fit 3-5 bell peppers, fill 3/4 full with water and bring to soft boil. Carefully place bell peppers in water and cook for about 10 minutes. They should be half way between crunchy and mushy. Don't cook them too long or they will become too soggy. Remove from water, rinse with cold water until completely cooled, this prevents further cooking; set aside.

Filling: Coat large skillet with non-stick cooking spray. Crumble and cook ground turkey, onion and celery over medium-high heat until turkey is cooked thoroughly and vegetables are tender. In large mixing bowl combine meat mixture, one can of tomato sauce and remaining ingredients, stir until well blended. If you desire a thicker tomato sauce mixture, add and additional 1/2-1 can of tomato sauce.

Spoon filling into bell peppers filling to the top. Place in shallow baking dish coated with non-stick cooking spray. Sprinkle with cheese if desired. Bake for 30-35 minutes. If tops are getting too brown, before baking time is complete, cover with foil and continue to bake until done. Serve with salad, an extra vegetable, or just as they are.

Side Dishes

Vegetable Side Dishes:
Pasta Primavera
Veggie Rice Cakes

Potato Side Dishes:
Mashed Potatoes
Baked Potato Splurge
Twice Baked Potatoes
French Fries

Salads:
Pasta Salad
Green Salad
Potato Salad

Vegetable Side Dishes

Pasta Primavera

Choose your own variety of vegetables. Select multi-colored vegetables to make this dish more attractive.

6-8 oz. Angel hair pasta *
2 Cups sliced mushrooms
1/2 Cup julienned carrots
1 Cup diced zucchini

1/2 Cup minced **shallots** or onion
1-2 Minced garlic cloves
1 tsp. Italian blend herbs

Begin to bring large pot of water to a boil for pasta. As water is heating begin to cook vegetables. Generously coat large skillet with non-stick cooking spray, heat over medium-high to high heat. When cooking surface is very hot add mushrooms and carrots. Cook for 4-5 minutes, turning frequently. Add remaining ingredients and cook an additional two minutes. Remove from heat. By now water should be boiling. Cook pasta for 2-4 minutes, drain. Put desired amount of pasta on plate and spoon vegetable mixture on top. Another option would be to toss the vegetables with the pasta and serve.

Note: If you choose to use chopped tomatoes, stir them in after you have removed the vegetables from the heat. This will warm them without overcooking.

* Angel hair pasta compliments this meal very nicely. Because of the pasta's thin shape, the flavor of the pasta does not overpower the flavor of the vegetables. Angel hair pasta is easy to find in beet (red), spinach (green) and regular (yellow) flavors. Mixing a variety of them together make a flavorful and attractive dish. Other pastas may substituted.

Alternative: Serve this dish as a main course by adding thin strips of cooked chicken or turkey breast or a side of fish.

Veggie Rice Cakes

These make a great and easy side dish for any meal. A real snap if you have leftover rice.

2 Cups brown rice, cooked, cooled	6-8 Egg whites
1 Cup grated zucchini	1/2 tsp. Garlic powder
1/2 Cup chopped green onion	1/2 tsp. Salt-free blend
1/2 Cup grated carrots	

In medium-sized mixing bowl blend together all ingredients. Batter should be thick. Coat large skillet or griddle with non-stick cooking spray, heat over medium-high heat. Spoon batter onto cooking surface making 2"-3" round cakes. Cook for 4-6 minutes on each side, until golden brown and firm.

Potato Side Dishes

Mashed Potatoes

8-10 Small baking potatoes, peeled and diced
1/2 Cup nonfat milk, warmed
1/2 Cup nonfat sour cream

Optional ingredients: 1/2 Cup evaporated skimmed milk
1 Packet *Butter Buds*, dry
1/4 Cup chopped chives
1/4 Cup chopped, green onions
1/4 Cup finely chopped turkey bacon or ham, cooked and cooled

Whenever I pulled the short straw and had to peel potatoes, it was mandatory to remove all the brown spots from each potato. I was told that this would make the potatoes more appealing to the eye. I'm not so careful any more. In fact, one time I didn't peel any of the potatoes, they were a little chewy, but nonetheless nutritious. The choice is yours.

Clean potatoes under running water making sure to remove any eyes (roots). Peel and cut potatoes into evenly sized pieces. The smaller the pieces the quicker they cook. Place in large pot covering with 2" of water. Bring to medium boil and continue to cook until potatoes are very tender, 20-30 minutes. Remove from heat, drain water and mash potatoes with potato masher, large fork or hand mixer. Add just enough liquid to moisten potatoes, whip with hand mixer until desired texture. The amount of liquid and addition of extra ingredients will vary depending on how much you are making.

Optional ingredients: Stir in onions, chives and chopped meat after potatoes are whipped.

Note: A hand mixer is not mandatory, a potato masher will work just fine. A hand mixer enables you to whip the potatoes for a creamier, fluffier texture. If potatoes turn out lumpy, this means you probably didn't cook the potatoes long enough.

Baked Potato Splurge

Every once in a while I have a craving for one of those big baked potatoes with sour cream, butter, chives and bacon bits. Since this really isn't an option, I created my own version of the ultimate baked potato.

Large russet baking potato(s)

Butter Buds made into liquid form
Nonfat sour cream, plus skim milk
Green onions, finely chopped

Fresh chives, finely chopped
Turkey bacon, chopped then cooked, (1 slice for 2 potatoes)

Preheat oven to 450 degrees.

Clean potatoes under running water making sure to remove any eyes (roots). Before baking, insert small knife into potato, one inch deep, 4-6 times around potato. Bake for 20 minutes, turn potato over, continue to bake until fork or knife easily slides in and out of potato, approximately another 20-25 minutes. The larger the potato the longer it will take to cook. You can microwave the potatoes but the texture of the potato and outer skin are a little different. I find oven-baked potatoes much more flavorable.

While potatoes are baking, evenly chop turkey bacon strips and cook in small frying pan until crisp. Place on paper towel; set aside.

Prepare *Butter Buds* as directed on the package for liquid form; set aside.

In small bowl, add as much sour cream as you think you'll be using. Add a teaspoon at a time of skim milk and stir until smooth. You can use the sour cream right from the container but I find it a little too thick.

Preparing potato: Split potato open by cutting a "+" in top of potato, pinch top of potato to expose pulp, or cut potato in half lengthwise. Pour in liquid *Butter Buds*, add sour cream, onions, chives and top with turkey bacon bits.

If you are serving these baked potatoes for a group of people it is fun to let everyone make their own. Put the condiments in small bowls with individual spoons that can be passed around the table. The liquid *Butter Buds* can be put in a small pitcher for easy pouring.

It may not be the real McCoy, but it does satisfy the craving.

Twice Baked Potatoes

4 Large baking potatoes, russet
1/2 Cup nonfat sour cream
1/4-1/2 Cup nonfat milk
3/4 Cup nonfat grated cheese
   plus 1/4 cup to sprinkle on top
1/3 Cup finely chopped, green onions
3 Strips turkey bacon, chopped and cooked crisp
2 Tbls. finely chopped fresh chives

Preheat oven to 450 degrees.

Clean potatoes under running water making sure to remove any eyes (roots). Before baking insert small knife into potato, one inch deep, 4-6 times. Bake for 20 minutes, turn potato over, continue baking until fork or knife easily slides in and out of potato, approximately another 20-25 minutes. The larger the potato the longer it will take to cook. You can microwave the potatoes but the texture of the potato and outer skin are a little different. I find oven-baked potatoes much more flavorable and the skins are more sturdy for this purpose.

Reduce oven temperature to 350 degrees. Cut each potato in half lengthwise, let cool for 10-15 minutes. With spoon, scrape cooked potato away from skins and put in a mixing bowl. Do your best not to tear the potato skin. Set aside potato skin boats.

Add sour cream and milk to potato mixture, blend together with hand mixer until smooth. Add more sour cream or skimmed milk if a creamier texture is desired. Stir in remaining ingredients. Generously spoon potato mixture back into potato skin boats. Place on cookie sheet or shallow baking dish and bake for 15-20 minutes. Five minutes before potatoes are done baking, sprinkle with additional grated cheese. Remove from oven and serve.

French Fries

Baking potatoes, medium (2 per person)
Non-stick cooking spray
Optional seasonings:
    Chili powder   Dill
    Garlic or onion powder   Cajun Blend
    No-salt blends

Preheat oven to 450 degrees.

Clean potatoes under running water making sure to remove any eyes (roots). Slice potatoes lengthwise into 1/2-3/4" sticks or cut into 1/2- 3/4" rounds. Place on plate, cover with paper towel and microwave for 7-10 minutes, until potatoes are tender, not crunchy. Don't stack potatoes too high on plate. If necessary, microwave two platefuls. Coat shallow pan with non-stick spray (cookie sheet or pizza pan will work well) spread potatoes evenly on pan, try not to overlap. Lightly spray potatoes with non-stick cooking spray. Sprinkle on herbs or spices, bake for 8-10 minutes, until brown. Turn potatoes and continue to bake an additional 8-10 minutes.

Alternative method: If you don't have a microwave, use leftover baked potatoes or bake some potatoes ahead of time specifically for this purpose (see below).

Clean potatoes under running water making sure to remove any eyes (roots). Before cooking insert small knife into potato, one inch deep, 4-6 times around potato. Bake for 30-45 minutes depending on size of potatoes. Allow potatoes to cool 15-20 minutes. Slice potatoes lengthwise into 1/2-3/4" pieces or cut into 1/2-3/4" round slices. Coat shallow pan with non-stick cooking spray (cookie sheet or pizza pan will work well) spread potatoes evenly on pan, try not to overlap. Lightly spray potatoes with non-stick cooking spray, sprinkle with herbs and spices if desired.

Place potatoes under broiler for 8-12 minutes, turning halfway through to brown evenly. If the top rack in your oven sits too close to the heating element, drop the rack down one level.

Salads

Pasta Salad

1 Pkg. **rainbow rottini pasta**, cooked, drained, cooled
1/2 Cup carrots thinly sliced, 1" sticks
1/2 Cup diced broccoli
1/2 Cup chopped bell pepper
1/2 Cup diced zucchini
1/2 Cup chopped green onions
1/2 Cup chopped water chestnuts
1-3 Cloves minced garlic
4-6 Strips turkey bacon, chopped
1/4 Cup fresh chopped **parsley**
Nonfat **Italian salad dressing**

Garnish: Sliced hard-boiled egg whites
Paprika
Parsley sprigs

Cook pasta according to instructions on package. If you prefer your pasta more firm, cook for two minutes less than maximum suggested cooking time. Drain; set aside to cool.

In large skillet coated with non-stick cooking spray, sauté carrots, broccoli, and bell peppers over medium-high heat for 7-10 minutes, or until vegetables begin to tenderize. Add next five ingredients and continue sautéing until turkey bacon is well done. Add parsley, cook for an additional minute then combine vegetable mixture with pasta, stir gently. Slowly, and gradually, add salad dressing, stirring to coat vegetables and pasta. Stop when everything is well coated. Don't drown the salad in dressing. Garnish with sliced egg whites, paprika and parsley sprigs.

Green Salad

Greens: Red leaf lettuce
         Spinach
         Romaine lettuce
         Butterhead lettuce
         Kale
         Cabbage

Fixins: Cucumbers, Celery, Carrots, Egg whites, Tuna, Sprouts, Croutons, Tomatoes, Onions, Broccoli, Chicken breast, Turkey breast, Jicama, Breadcrumbs

Salad Dressings: Lemon/herb
    Vinaigrette
    Low/nonfat dressings in moderation

Clean and dry greens. Cut or break into bit-sized pieces, put into large bowl or on individual salad plates. Garnish with your choice of fixins. Toss if salad is in bowl. Serve with dressings "on the side" so each person can control amount of dressing. Use just enough dressing to add flavor, do not drown your salad, save yourself the calories.

Potato Salad

6 Cups diced red potatoes (6-8 potatoes), unpeeled
1/4 Cup chopped ham or turkey bacon
1/2 Cup chopped dill or sweet pickles
1/4 Cup chopped celery leaves (optional)
4 Hard-boiled egg whites, chopped
1 tsp. Italian herb blend
1/2 Cup nonfat sour cream
1/2 Cup nonfat mayonnaise
1 Tbls. Dijon mustard
1/2 Cup chopped celery
1/4 Cup chopped green onion

Clean and dice potatoes into 1 1/2" -2" pieces, put in large pot and cover with 2" of water. Bring water to medium boil for 20-25 minutes. Start checking for tenderness at fifteen minute mark. Drain and let cool. Cook ham or turkey bacon until light brown, set aside. In large mixing bowl combine remaining ingredients, stir gently. Add potatoes and ham or turkey bacon, stir until well blended. Serve warm or chilled.

Appetizers

Famous Layered Bean Dip

Potato Skin Appetizers

Famous Layered Bean Dip

Anybody who has ever been to a large gathering of friends, family, co-workers and the like, has dipped a chip or two into a wonderfully tasty layered bean dip. Here is how to prepare and eat it without guilt.

1/2 lb. Lean ground turkey breast	1/2 Cup chopped tomatoes
1/2 Small pkt. taco seasonings plus, 1/4 cup water	1/2 Cup chopped green onions
1 - 15 oz. can nonfat refried beans	1-2 Bags no-oil (baked) tortilla chips, plain or seasoned, unsalted
1 - 4 oz. can diced green chilies	Fresh salsa
1 Cup nonfat sour cream	

Spray skillet with non-stick cooking spray, heat over medium-high heat. Crumble turkey into skillet and cook until turkey is completely cooked. Reduce heat to medium-low, add taco seasoning and water, stir until well blended and water is evaporated. Remove from heat and let cool.

Heat refried beans in sauce pan or microwave. In 9" deep dish (pie plate, cake pan, baking dish) evenly spread refried beans. In order, evenly layer seasoned ground turkey breast, green chilies, sour cream, tomatoes and green onions. Serve with chips and salsa.

To serve dip warm, layer as above omitting sour cream and tomatoes. Bake at 375 degrees for 20 minutes, remove from oven. Evenly sprinkle on chopped tomatoes and serve. The sour cream can be a side dip, along with the fresh salsa

Alternative: Serve with warmed tortillas. Spoon dip onto tortilla and roll.

Potato Skin Appetizers

4 Small to medium baking potatoes
4-5 Slices turkey bacon or minced ham
1 Cup nonfat shredded cheese
2 Tbls. finely chopped **chives**
1/4 Cup finely chopped green onion
Nonfat sour cream, to top

Preheat oven to 450 degrees.

Clean potatoes under running water making sure to remove any eyes (roots). Before baking insert small knife into potato, one inch deep 4-6 times around potato. Bake for 15-20 minutes then turn potatoes over, continue baking until fork or knife easily slides in and out of potato, approximately another 15-20 minutes. The larger the potato the longer it will take to cook. To save time, microwave the potatoes, however, I find oven-baked potatoes much more flavorable and the skins are more sturdy for this purpose.

Reduce oven temperature to 350 degrees. Cut each potato in half lengthwise, let cool for 10-15 minutes. With spoon scrape cooked potato away from skins, leaving approximately 1/4" - 1/2" of pulp. Put excess potato pulp in an air tight container and use for mashed potatoes or breakfast potatoes. Be careful not to tear the potato skin. Place potato skin boat on cookie sheet, lightly coat inside of shell with non-stick cooking spray. Bake in oven for 8-10 minutes or until boats become crisp. Remove from oven; set aside.

Chop turkey bacon slices in to small 1/4" pieces. Cook bacon or ham in small skillet over medium heat until crisp. Let cool. Evenly sprinkle cheese into potato skin boats, place in oven for 3-5 minutes to melt and brown cheese. Remove from oven and sprinkle ham or bacon bits, chives and green onions into boats. Add a dollop of sour cream, if desired, and enjoy the show/game.

Desserts

Pumpkin Cookies

Peach Cobbler

Strawberry Shortcake

Fruit Glaze

Pumpkin Cookies

1 Cup whole wheat flour
1/3 Cup of sugar or equivalent
 amount of artificial sweetener *
1 1/2 tsp. Ground cinnamon
1/2 tsp. Allspice
1/2 Cup oats

1 tsp. Baking powder
1/4 tsp. Baking soda
3/4 Cup mashed, cooked pumpkin
1/4 Cup unsweetened applesauce
2 Egg whites
1/4 Cup raisins (optional)

* See equivalents on sweetener product you choose to use.

Preheat oven to 375 degrees. Coat cookie sheet with non-stick cooking spray.

In medium size mixing bowl, combine dry ingredients (first 7). In small mixing bowl combine pumpkin, applesauce, egg whites and raisins. Add to dry ingredients and stir just until dry ingredients are moistened. Spoon batter onto cookie sheet making 2 inch circles. Bake for 15-17 minutes.

For an extra large batch:

2 2/3 Cup whole wheat flour
1 Cup oats
1 Cup sugar or equivalent
 amount of artificial sweetener *
1 Tbls. cinnamon
1 tsp. Allspice

2 tsp. Baking powder
1 tsp. Baking soda
2 Cups mashed, cooked pumpkin
1/2 Cup raisins (optional)
1/2 Cup unsweetened applesauce
5 Egg whites

* See equivalents on sweetener product you choose to use.

Prepare as instructed above.

Peach Cobbler

Strawberry and rhubarb, raspberries, blackberries, blueberries and baking apples can be used in this versatile cobbler recipe. This recipe can easily be doubled.

3 Cups peaches, peeled and sliced
1/2 Cup unsweetened apple juice concentrate, undiluted
2 Tbls. tapioca or cornstarch

1/4 tsp. Cinnamon
1/3 + 1/2 Cup reduced fat biscuit mix
1/3 Cup nonfat milk

Preheat oven to 350 degrees. Coat 8" x 8" baking dish with non-stick cooking spray.

Peel peaches with potato peeler or blanch in very hot water (low boil) for 3-4 minutes to easily remove skins. Slice into medium-sized mixing bowl. Add tapioca, fruit juice and cinnamon, stir until well blended. If you are using cornstarch, place cornstarch in small cup, gradually add fruit juice stirring quickly. Stir until corn starch mixture is smooth. Add to peaches with cinnamon, blend well. Pour fruit mixture into baking dish.

In small bowl combine biscuit mix and milk. Drop small spoonfuls of biscuit batter on top of fruit. Biscuits will enlarge during baking, be sure to disperse evenly without overlapping.

Bake for 25-30 minutes until biscuits are golden brown and fruit is bubbly. Let cool, serve.

Strawberry Shortcake

This shortcake doesn't have to be made strictly with strawberries. Try apples, peaches, blueberries, blackberries, raspberries, or bananas.

Shortcake:
- 2 Cups reduced fat biscuit mix
- 3/4 Cup nonfat milk
- 1/2 tsp. Cinnamon

Fruit Glaze:
- 1 - 12 oz. Can Unsweetened fruit juice, undiluted
   (Apple juice seems to suit most fruits)
- 2 Tbls. cornstarch

2-3 Pints strawberries (or 2-4 Cups of fruit of your choice)

Preheat oven to 450 degrees. Clean strawberries and remove tops. Cut in half and place in bowl. Make fruit glaze, let cool (See Fruit Glaze recipe). Combine biscuit mix and milk. Spoon batter onto ungreased cookie sheet making 7-9 shortcakes. Bake for 8-10 minutes or until golden brown. Remove from oven, let cool.

Add 1/2 cup of fruit glaze, at a time, to fruit until you have desired consistency. Split shortcakes in half, lay halves in serving bowl or on small plate. If you have leftover glaze, spread one teaspoon over each shortcake half. Spoon fruit over shortcake halves and serve.

Alternative: Spread a layer of nonfat cream cheese on shortcake halves before topping with fruit.

Fruit Glaze

Apple juice concentrate is the most versatile flavored juice. It compliments most dishes it is used in.

1-16 oz. Can unsweetened fruit juice concentrate, undiluted, thawed
3 Tbls. corn starch
OR
1-12 oz. Can unsweetened fruit juice concentrate, undiluted, thawed
2 Tbls. corn starch

Place corn starch in measuring cup or small bowl. Slowly add approximately 1/2 can fruit juice, stirring quickly until well blended and lump-free. Pour rest of fruit juice in small sauce pan, cook over medium-high heat to a slow boil. Stir in corn starch mixture, stirring constantly until glaze begins to thicken. Stir until desired thickness is reached, remove from heat, let cool

Alternatives: If a thicker glaze is desired add an additional 1/2 tsp. of cornstarch per four ounces of juice; 1 1/2 tsp. for a 12 oz. can of juice, and 2 tsp. for a 16 oz. can. To make fruit syrup, use 1 Tbls. plus 1 tsp. of cornstarch for a 12 oz. can of juice, and 2 Tbls. plus 1 tsp. of cornstarch for a 16 oz. can.

Bibliography

Dunne, Lavon J. Nutrition Almanac, Third Edition. McGraw-Hill, 1990

Herbst, Sharon Tyler. Food Lover's Companion. Hauppauge, New York. Barrons Educational Series, 1990

Martin, Kimberly and Martin, Dennis. Espresso Magic, sixth edition. Lake Forest Park, Washington, Shady Lane Enterprises

A

Aerobic exercise, 55, 57-58
  See also Exercise
  calculating target heart rate, 57-58
Alcoholic beverages, 35
Appetizers, 11, 64, 121-123
  potato skins, 64, 123
  layered bean dip, 64, 122
Applejuice, 19, 128
Apples, 18, 26, 127
Applesauce, 18, 27, 41
Artery disorders, 51
Arthritis, 6
Artificial sweeteners, 20, 33, 41
Avocado, 8, 35, 43

B

Bacon, 8, 35
  See also Turkey bacon
Bagels, 6, 22, 42, 60
Baking Hints, 41
Baking Spices, 19
Bananas, 18, 26, 127
Barbecue beef sandwich, 61, 87
Barbecue chicken breast sandwich, 61
Barbecue pork sandwich, 61, 87
Barbecue sauce, 13, 19, 33 60
Barley, 5, 88
Bean dip, layered, 64, 122
Beans, 6, 18, 29, 62
Beef, 6, 8, 17, 23, 36
  boneless ribs, 17, 62, 93
  broth, 18, 30
  eye of round, 17, 24, 38, 62, 93
  loins, 23, 38
  London broil, 17, 24, 62
  rounds, 23, 38
  sirloin, 38
  stew, 17, 62, 93
  stroganoff, 62
  tenderloin, 38
  top round, 38
Bell Peppers, 18, 27, 60
  stuffed, 60, 63, 111
Berries, 18, 26, 64, 127
Biscuit mix, 20, 34
Boboli, 107
Bread, 5, 14, 17, 38, 42
  bagels, 6, 17, 22, 42
  burger buns, 6, 17, 22
  pizza shell, 6, 17, 107
  sandwich, 44
  side dish, 44
  whole wheat, 17, 22, 38
Breadcrumbs, 20, 34
Breakfast, 42, 43, 60, 68-78
Broccoli, 18, 60
Broths, 18, 30, 39
Brunch, 60, 68-78
Bulgur, 5

Burger buns, 6, 17, 22
Burgers, 44
  turkey, 62
Burritos, 61, 104
  breakfast, 60, 75
Butter, 8, 13, 36, 39, 41
Butter Buds, 20, 34, 39
Buttermilk, 36

C

Cabbage, 18, 28
  stuffed rolls, 63, 110
Caffeine, 36, 51
Cake, 36, 39
Calories, 9-10, 58
Canadian bacon, 26, 60, 61
Candy, 13, 14, 36, 39
Carbohydrates, 5-6, 7, 9, 10
  refined, 5-6
Carrots, 18, 27
Casserole, chili, 60, 61, 63, 100
Catsup, 13, 19
Celery, 18, 28, 60
Cereal, 5, 14, 18, 29, 61
  cold, 18, 29, 61
  hot, 18, 29, 61, 71
  multi-grain, 71
  oats, 18, 71
  whole-grain, 18, 71
Cheese, 6, 8, 36, 38
  cottage, 17, 23, 64
  grated, 17
  hard, 23
Chicken, 6, 17, 25, 45
  barbecue chicken breast sandwich, 61
  breast, 25, 61, 62
  broth, 18, 30
  canned chunk light, 17, 26
  salad sandwich, 61, 86
  soup, 44, 61, 87
  stroganoff, 62, 94
Chili, 60, 61, 62, 98
  chili casserole, 60, 61, 63, 100
  turkey chili, 98-99
Chips, 14, 19, 39, 45, 62, 64
Chocolate, 8, 36, 51, 54
Cholesterol, 7, 55
Clam chowder, 44, 61, 89
Coffee, 3, 11
  See also Espresso Drinks
  caffeinated, 36
  decaffeinated, 51-53
  whole bean, 51
Condiments, 13, 14, 15
  See also specific condiment
Cookies, 13, 14, 36, 39
Corn, 5, 18, 28
Cornmeal, 20, 34
Crock pot dinners, 62, 92-93
  boneless beef spareribs, 62, 93

boneless pork spareribs, 62, 92
eye of round beef roast, 62, 93
pork loin roast, 62, 92
stewed beef, 62, 93
turkey breast, 62, 92
turkey breast tenderloins, 62, 92
Croissants, 36
Croutons, 32

D
Dairy products, 6, 8, 17, 38
   See also Cheese
   See also Eggs
   See also Milk
   half-n-half, 36, 38
   sour cream, 36, 38, 72
   whipping cream, 36, 38
Decaffeinated, 51-53
Desserts, 46, 64, 124-128
   fruit glaze, 38, 41, 128
   peach cobbler, 64, 126
   pumpkin cookies, 64, 125
   strawberry shortcake, 64, 127
Diabetes, 6
Dinner, 45-46, 62-63, 66, 90-111
Doughnuts, 36
Dressing, See also Stuffing
   salad, 8, 13, 19, 36, 40
Duck, 45

E
Eating, 8-9, 11, 55-56
   how much, 8-9, 55-56
   when, 8, 55-56
Egg and tuna sandwich, 86
Eggs, 6, 8, 17, 23, 38, 40, 41, 42, 60
   egg hash, 60, 75
   omelettes, 42, 60, 73
   scrambled, 60, 74
   substitutes, 17, 40, 41, 42
   toppings, 60, 72
   yolks, 23, 36, 43, 72
Egg salad sandwich, 23, 61, 86
Eggs Benedict, 42
Espresso drinks, 3, 51-54
Exercise, 8, 9, 55, 57-58
   aerobic, 55, 57-58
   weight training, 55, 57-58

F
Fajitas, 63
Fat free, 2, 9
Fats, 7, 9, 10, 12
Fish, 7, 17, 25, 45-46, 62
Flour, 6, 41
   tortillas, 6, 19, 32
   whole-wheat, 6, 20, 22
Food Substitutes, 3, 38
French fries, 46, 63, 118
French toast, 22, 43, 60, 69

Frozen yogurt, 36
Fruit, 5, 13, 18, 26, 64
   See also specific fruit
   glaze, 38, 41, 128
   juice, 11, 19, 33, 128
   popsicles, 13, 19, 64
   spreads, 20, 27, 39, 42, 43
Fruit Glaze, 38, 41, 128

G
Gaining weight, 2, 8, 9, 10, 55-56
Garlic, 18, 27
Grains, 5
Grapes, 18
Gravy, 22, 92, 93
Green chilies, 19, 31, 72
Green leaf lettuce, 18
Grocery List, Master, 17-20
Grocery shopping, 2, 15, 16

H
Half-n-half, 36, 38
Ham, 24, 26, 60, 61
Heart aggravations, 51
Heartburn, 51
Herbs, 19
Honey, 36, 41
Hypertension, 51
Hypoglycemia, 51
Hypothyroidism, 51

I
Ice Cream, 13, 14, 36, 39
Insomnia, 51
Italian dishes, 63, 106-109
   lasagna, 61, 63, 106
   manicotti, 63, 109
   pizza, 61, 63, 107
   quick and easy spaghetti meat sauce, 108
   spaghetti meat sauce, 108

K
Kebabs, 62, 95
Ketchup SEE Catsup

L
Label reading, 7, 9
Lasagna, 61, 63, 106
Legumes, 6
Lunch, 43-45, 61-62, 66, 85-89
Lunch meat, 17, 26, 36

M
Manicotti, 60, 63, 109
Maple extract, 19
Maple syrup, 71
Margarine, 8, 36, 39, 41
Marinade, 39, 40
Marinara, 18, 46, 72
Mayonnaise, 8, 13, 19, 32, 36, 38

Meat, 6, 17, 38, 45
  See also Beef
  See also Chicken
  See also Pork
  See also Turkey
  breakfast, 43
  lunch, 17, 26, 36
Meatballs, 23, 62, 97
Meatloaf, 23, 61, 62, 97
Menu ideas, 2, 3, 59-64
  appetizers, 64
  breakfast, 60-61
  brunch, 60-61
  desserts, 64
  dinner, 62-63
  lunch, 61-62
  side dishes, 63-64
  snacks, 64
Metabolism, 1, 6, 8-9, 58
Mexican dishes, 63, 101-105
  burritos, 61, 63, 104
  fajitas, 63
  nachos, 105
  quesadilla, 63, 101
  soft tacos, 63, 103
  tostadas, 63, 102
Milk, 6, 11, 14, 17, 22, 36, 38
  2%, 36, 38
  dry, powdered, 17
  evaporated, skim, 17, 22, 38
  nonfat, 17, 22, 38
  whole, 36, 38
Mineral depletion, 6
Molasses, 35
Muffins, 22, 60, 64, 79-84
  banana blueberry, 83
  banana cornmeal, 81, 99, 100
  blueberry, 84
  cinnamon apple, 80
  pumpkin bran, 82
Muscles, 55, 57-58
  atrophy, 1, 57
  growth, 6, 55, 57
  meats,7
Mushrooms, 18, 28, 60
Mustard, 19

N
Nachos, 105
Non-stick cooking spray, 20, 39
No-salt blends, 38
Nut butters, 8, 35
Nuts, 6, 8, 35, 43

O
Oats, 5, 29, 71
Obesity, 6
Oils, 8, 35, 41
  vegetable, 35, 39
Olives, 8, 35, 43

Omelettes, 42, 60, 73
  Philly-style steak, 74
Onions, 18, 27, 60
Osteoporosis, 57

P
Pancakes, 40, 43, 60, 69, 70
  mix, 20, 34
  rice, 40, 60, 70
Pasta, 5, 19, 31, 46, 63
  manicotti, 63
  primavera, 63, 113
  salad, 44, 62, 119
Pastries, 36
Peach cobbler, 126
Peaches, 18, 26, 127
Pears, 18
Philly-style omelette, 74
Philly-style steak sandwich, 61, 87
Pickles, 13, 19
  relish, 19, 33
Pies, 36, 39
Pineapple, 18, 27
Pizza, 61, 63, 107
Polynesian sauce, 95-96
Pork, 6, 17, 24, 38, 62, 92
  boneless spareribs, 17, 62, 92
  chops, 17, 62, 92
  ham, 17, 24, 26, 60, 61
  loin roast, 17, 24, 62, 92
Popcorn, 5, 8, 13, 19, 64
Popsicles, 13, 19, 64
Portions, 9, 10, 11
Potatoes, 5, 18, 28, 29, 42, 46, 60, 63
  baked potato splurge, 63, 116
  breakfast, 42, 60, 78
  diced, 60, 63, 78
  French fries, 46, 63, 118
  fried mashed, 60, 63, 78
  hash browns, 60, 78
  mashed, 22, 46, 66, 115
  potato skin appetizer, 63, 123
  salad, 44, 120
  twice baked, 63, 117
Poultry, 6, 24-26, 45
  See also Chicken
  See also Duck
  See also Turkey
Preparation Alternatives, 40
Pretzels, 13, 19, 64
Produce, 18, 26-28
  See also specific fruit
  See also specific vegetable
Protein, 5, 6, 7, 9, 10
Pumpkin, 19, 30, 54
  cookies, 64, 125
  porridge, 22, 61, 71

Q
Quesadilla, 63, 64, 101

Quiche, 60, 77
Quick and Easy Spaghetti Meat Sauce, 108

R
Raisins, 18, 26
Reading labels, 7, 9
Recipes, 65-128
   appetizers, 121-123
   breakfast/brunch, 68-78
   desserts, 124-128
   dinner, 90-111
   lunch, 85-89
   muffins, 79-84
   side dishes, 112-120
Refried beans, 18, 30
Relish, 19, 33
Restaurant dining, 37, 42-50
Restaurant Food Choices, 42-46
Restaurant menu items, 47-50
Rice, 5, 19, 32, 40, 46, 63
   brown, 19, 32, 63
   rice pancakes, 32, 60, 70
   veggie rice cakes, 63, 114
Rye, 5

S
Salad, 43, 44, 45, 64, 119-120
   coleslaw, 44, 64
   fruit, 44, 62, 64
   green leaf, 43, 62, 64, 120
   pasta, 44, 62, 119
   potato, 44, 120
Salad dressing, 8, 13, 19, 36, 40
Salami, 36
Salsa, 19, 33, 60, 64, 72
Salt SEE Sodium
Sandwiches, 22, 44, 61, 86-87
   barbecue beef, 61, 87
   barbecue chicken breast, 61
   barbecue pork, 61, 87
   chicken salad, 61, 86
   egg and tuna salad, 61, 86
   egg salad, 61, 86
   French dip, 61
   fried egg and ham, 61
   Philly-style steak, 61, 87
   tuna salad, 61, 86
   turkey salad, 61, 86
Sausage, 8, 36, 42, 47
Sautéing, 40
Seafood, 6, 7, 17, 36
   See also Fish or Shellfish
Seasoning packets, 13, 19, 40
Seasonings, SEE Spices
Shellfish, 7, 36
Shortening, 8, 36, 41
Side dishes, 112-120
   baked potato splurge, 63, 116
   French fries, 46, 63, 118
   green salad, 43, 62, 64, 120

   mashed potatoes, 115
   pasta primavera, 113
   pasta salad, 44, 62, 119
   potato salad, 44, 120
   stuffing/dressing, 19, 32, 63
   twice baked potatoes, 63, 117
   vegetables, 64
   veggie rice cakes, 63, 114
Snacks, 13, 14, 19, 64
Soda pop, 11, 36
Sodium, 10, 13, 36, 38, 40, 41
Soft tacos, 63, 103
Soups, 36, 44, 45, 88-89
   chicken, 44, 61, 88
   clam chowder, 44, 61, 89
   cream, 22
   turkey, 44, 61, 88
   vegetable beef, 44, 61, 87
Sour cream, nonfat 6, 17, 23, 72
Soybean products, 6, 36
Spaghetti sauce, 18, 60, 61, 63, 108
Spices, 19
Spinach, 18, 28, 60, 64
Squash, 18
   See also Zucchini
Strawberry shortcake, 64, 127
String beans, 18
Stroganoff, 62, 94
   beef, 62, 94
   chicken, 94
   turkey, 62, 94
Stuffed bell peppers, 60, 63,111
Stuffed cabbage rolls, 63, 110
Stuffing/dressing, 19, 32, 63
Sugars, 5, 6, 10, 13, 36, 41
   health risks, 6
Sunflower seeds, 36, 43
Syrup, 20, 34, 38
   sugar free, 20, 34

T
Tapioca, 20, 34
Tartar sauce, 33
Tea, 11, 51
Toast, 22, 42, 60
Tomatoes, 18, 60
   chunky sauce, 18
   juice, 19
   paste, 18, 30
   sauce, 18, 30
   stewed, 18, 30
Toppings for egg dishes, 60, 72
Tortillas, 5, 6, 19, 32
Tostada, 63, 102
   breakfast, 60, 76
Tuna, canned, 17, 26
   albacore, 26
   chunk light, 17, 26
Tuna salad sandwich, 86
Turkey, 6, 17, 25, 45

See also Turkey, ground breast
bacon, 17
salad sandwich, 61, 86
smoked turkey breast, 17, 25, 61
soup, 44, 61, 88
stroganoff, 62, 94
tenderloins, 17, 25, 92
whole breast, 17, 25, 92
Turkey, ground breast, 17, 24, 38, 60
   burgers, 62
   burritos, 104
   chili, 60, 61, 62, 98
   chili casserole, 60, 61, 63, 100
   egg hash, 60, 75
   manicotti, 63, 109
   meatballs, 97
   meatloaf, 97
   nachos, 105
   stuffed bell peppers, 111
   stuffed cabbage rolls, 110
   tacos, 103

U
Ulcer, 51

V
Vanilla extract, 19
Vegetables, 5, 18, 27, 46, 64
   See also specific vegetable
   beef soup, 44, 61, 87
   broth, 18, 30
   cooking spray, SEE Non-Stick Cooking Spray
   oil, 35, 39
Vegetable dishes, 63, 110-111, 113-114
   See also Salads
   pasta primavera, 63, 113
   stuffed bell peppers, 63, 111
   stuffed cabbage rolls, 63, 110
   veggie rice cakes, 63, 114

W
Waffles, 40, 43, 60, 69
Water chestnuts, 19, 31
Weight gain, 2, 8, 9, 10, 55-56
Weight gain drink, 22, 23, 56
Whole-grain flour, 6
Whole wheat, 5
   bread, 6
   flour, 6, 20, 22, 41
   pancake mix, 6, 20, 34
   tortillas, 6
Wondra, 20, 34

Y
Yogurt, 6, 8, 17, 23, 54, 64
   frozen, 36

Z
Zucchini, 60, 95

Eat to be Lean: A Step-by-Step Guide to a Healthy Eating Lifestyle!

Yes! I would like to share this book with someone I care about. Please send me _____ copies of **Eat to be Lean: A Step-by-Step Guide to a Healthy Eating Lifestyle**. Please add an additional $2.95 per book, for postage and handling.

Quantity		Price Each	Total Due
	Eat to be Lean	$15.95	
		Subtotal:	
	WA Residents Only - Add 8.2% Sales Tax:		
		Postage and Handling:	
		Grand Total:	

Make check, money order or cashiers checks payable to: Mainstream Publishing
Mail to: Mainstream Publishing, P.O. Box 1252, Snohomish, WA 98291
Note: All out of country orders must be accompanied by a Postal Money order in U.S. funds.

Please allow 4-6 weeks for delivery.
Money Back Guarantee

I understand that if I am not completely satisfied with **Eat to be Lean: A Step-by-Step Guide to a Healthy Eating Lifestyle**, I may return the undamaged book, at my expense, within 10 days for a complete refund of the purchase price.

Eat to be Lean: A Step-by-Step Guide to a Healthy Eating Lifestyle!

Yes! I would like to share this book with someone I care about. Please send me _____ copies of **Eat to be Lean: A Step-by-Step Guide to a Healthy Eating Lifestyle**. Please add an additional $2.95 per book, for postage and handling.

Quantity		Price Each	Total Due
	Eat to be Lean	$15.95	
		Subtotal:	
	WA Residents Only - Add 8.2% Sales Tax:		
		Postage and Handling:	
		Grand Total:	

Make check, money order or cashiers checks payable to: Mainstream Publishing
Mail to: Mainstream Publishing, P.O. Box 1252, Snohomish, WA 98291
Note: All out of country orders must be accompanied by a Postal Money order in U.S. funds.

Please allow 4-6 weeks for delivery.
Money Back Guarantee

I understand that if I am not completely satisfied with **Eat to be Lean: A Step-by-Step Guide to a Healthy Eating Lifestyle**, I may return the undamaged book, at my expense, within 10 days for a complete refund of the purchase price.